Are you in pain, feeling helpless, lonely, stressed, "out of control," sad, confused, afraid, anxious, angry, lost, tired, frustrated, different, restless, overwhelmed, hopeless ... maybe even a combination of these? YOU ARE NOT ALONE!

Your pain is real. We know that. And there are many young people out there (right now) facing similar challenges. The interesting thing is ... your pain may actually be a sign of your strengths that you can use to change your well-being.

Bright. Creative. Sensitive. Observant. Perfectionist.

Is this you? *We see you.* And this book can help.

There is a way out of this dark hole of pain, and it starts with YOU. This book is about understanding how your brain works and using the resources you already have (like your brain!) to help alleviate suffering.

This book alone won't make your pain go away. But, as you work with your health team it will guide you to use tools that have been proven to help smart brain people like yourself. We will show you how your own strengths and efforts will make traditional and complementary mind-body therapies work more effectively to get you where you want to be.

You are more powerful than you may think ... Start reading to learn how you can "unstick" your own pain neural loops and move on to the life you want to live!

The Smart Brain Pain Syndrome

The Primer for Teens & Young Adults in Pain

Georgia Weston, LCSW
Lonnie K. Zeltzer, MD
Paul M. Zeltzer, MD

Creative Healing for Youth in Pain (CHYP)
www.mychyp.org

For information regarding permission,
please send an email to *admin@mychyp.org*.

DEDICATION

This book is dedicated to all the volunteers of Creative Healing for Youth in Pain (CHYP): past, present, and future. Your hard work, passion, and creativity are what fuel the organization and bring such powerful programs to our youth and families looking for help. Thank you for all that you do, not only for our team, but also for the community we serve together.

We give special recognition to the years of effort from Olivia, Laura, Sara, Shelley, Samantha, Liz, and Dana. CHYP would not be where it is today if it weren't for your generosity of time and spirit. We appreciate you and so do our families!

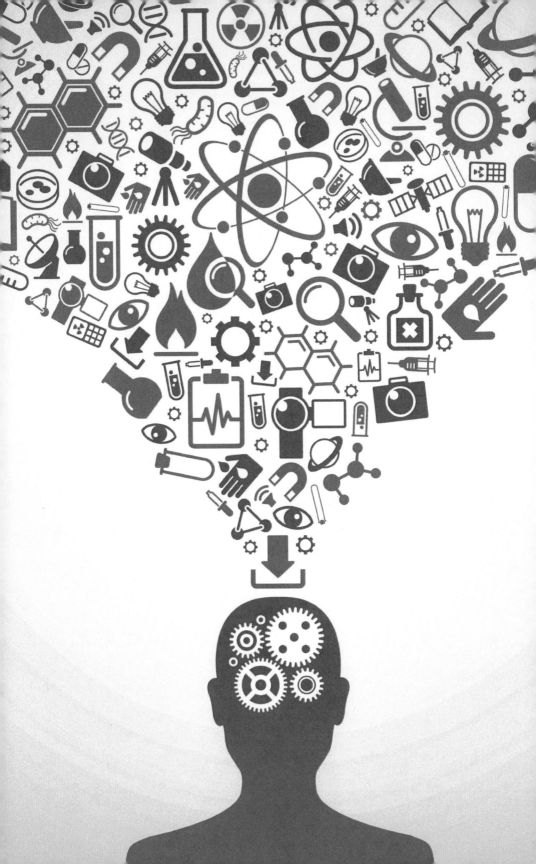

Preface: Who are We?

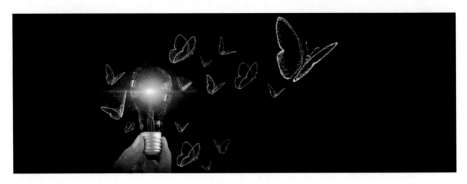

Who are "we"?

"We" is used a lot in this book, so we want to introduce ourselves. To put it simply, we are three people working together to help children, teens, and young adults solve the mystery of chronic pain. We each stumbled into this world of childhood chronic pain from different directions, and this book is a compilation of our observations, experiences, and unique perspectives on this healing journey. We'll each tell you a bit about ourselves here, and if you want to learn more about us, look at our full bios in the back of the book.

I'm Georgia Weston, LCSW, a chronic pain survivor and advocate. I was diagnosed with chronic pain at age 14. My diagnosis came only after visiting more than 20 doctors, countless emergency rooms, and a very scary ambulance ride. Most people thought I was faking it—that I was making up the pain for attention. I even started to doubt myself and referred to it as my "fake pain." I thought I was going crazy!

The whole process was hard—harder than it had to be. But I was lucky enough to be going through it in the 21st century, in Los Angeles, with health insurance and parents who could take the time to drive me to all my appointments. I had never heard of chronic pain, and I didn't know anyone my age who had it. The journey was terrifying and difficult, and the worst part for me was feeling alone. That's why I've dedicated my life to helping others through this confusing and lonely chronic pain maze. A combination of art, Iyengar yoga, and hypnotherapy is what helped me—but creative healing means different things for each person. It is about finding what works best for you!

I'm Dr. Lonnie Zeltzer, a pediatric chronic pain physician. I've been treating children who suffer from chronic pain for more than forty years. Over the decades I've noticed a clear pattern in my patients. Almost everyone who walks into my office is bright, sensitive, observant ... and usually a perfectionist. My patients have creative, intellectual minds—which is a good thing, but also can be adding "fuel to the fire" when it comes to pain. The brain is a fascinating instrument that truly has a mind of its own. An explanation of how brains experience and learn from pain is the most empowering gift I can give these young people. My patients have seen multiple doctors, undergone numerous tests, and taken many medications with no end to their pain. It became clear to me that a better approach was needed.

Most physicians are <u>not</u> taught how to treat chronic pain. I've learned to encourage a "creative healing" approach involving education, non-traditional healing options, and a supportive social environment. This book is step one: *education.* You have to know and understand what is happening to both your brain and body. That takes work, and this book is a great start.

I'm Dr. Paul Zeltzer, and I found my way into the pediatric chronic pain field after decades of working with children and teens with cancer who have acute pain. I am a neuro-oncologist, educator, brain cancer researcher, author, and entrepreneur; my medical career spans 40 years. Most of my efforts had been in the field of cancer-related pain, but chronic pain is more complicated and has to be addressed in a different way. I love meeting and working with children and teens who develop resilience right before me. I find it invigorating, because once they overcome this pain *thing,* a much deeper understanding of the preciousness of health develops. These young people gain a real sense of value from their experience. It's a gratifying adventure for everyone involved ... even if you didn't want it.

This book will explain many concepts, including the bio-psycho-social model. Each topic is important, but your **focus** here is on things **you** (the reader) can control.

As a final thought, we thank you for being curious enough to read this. Being open to learning is a skill that will take you far in life. So, let your interest blossom, make your own judgements about our words, and then create your own solutions that fit into your life.

Chapter 1: The Smart Brain Pain Syndrome

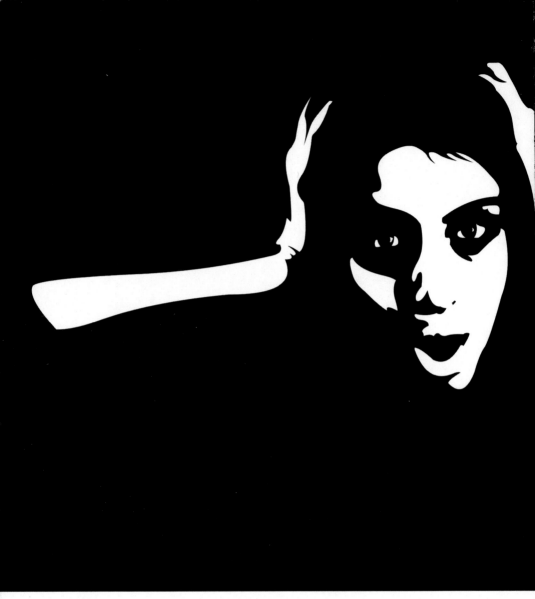

1a. Pain—How do we recognize it?

You know what it's like to feel pain. We've all had a paper cut or stubbed a toe, banged our "funny bone," or even held that hair dryer a little too close. We try to avoid it as best we can, but pain happens. It's a part of life.

Some people may wonder why we even need pain—*who wants that kind of discomfort?*

2

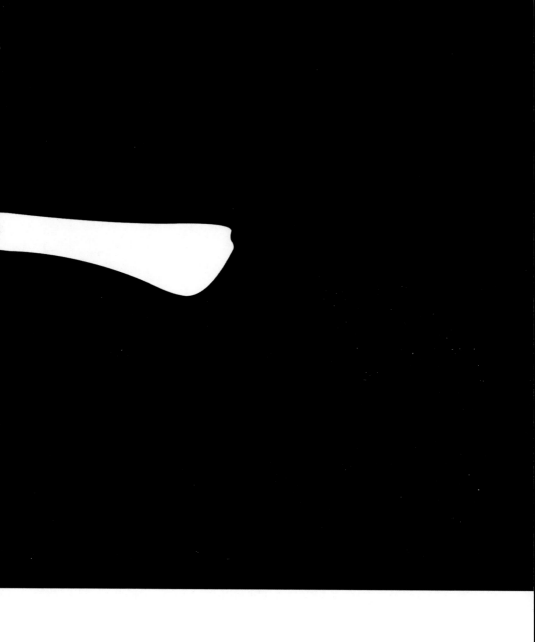

Well, believe it or not, from an evolutionary and survival perspective, pain *protects* us.

You may be wondering ... do we have to experience paper cuts? *Do we really need to be "protected" from paper?* Well, the simple answer is: yes.

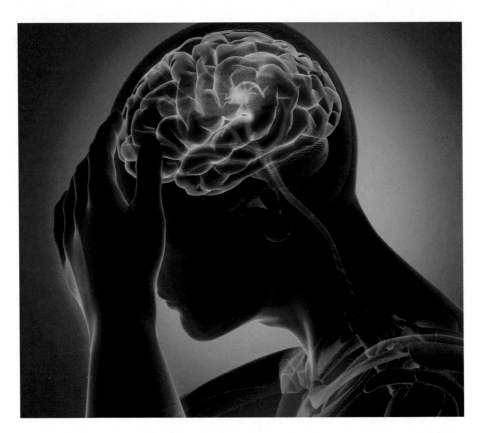

When we get paper cuts, as tiny as they are, they damage our skin. That wound exposes us to hazards like bacteria. We don't want them inside our bodies because they can lead to infection. So, when the paper breaks through the surface of our skin, we feel pain. Our brains are reminding us to be more careful—*let's not do that again.*

Obviously, a paper cut is a simple example, but we're just warming up here. Let's move it up a notch. Think about a time that you stubbed your toe. *It hurt.*

Again, the pain makes you think, "Let's not do that again." So, to avoid this same discomfort next time, your brain *learns*—walk a little slower, turn on the hallway light next time, or don't text while walking. Whichever reason your brain labels as "why" you stubbed your toe prior to the pain, **it automatically makes a note that you don't want to repeat this behavior.** It's a *Post-It* note in your brain—next time you'll avoid those actions and you won't stub your toe!

Pain can get a little more complicated though. In fact, there are two types of pain: "acute" and "chronic."

The examples we gave before fall under the category of acute pain. An injury happens, it heals, and it goes away—something everyone deals with. Since we're comparing acute pain with chronic pain, let's use some more examples.

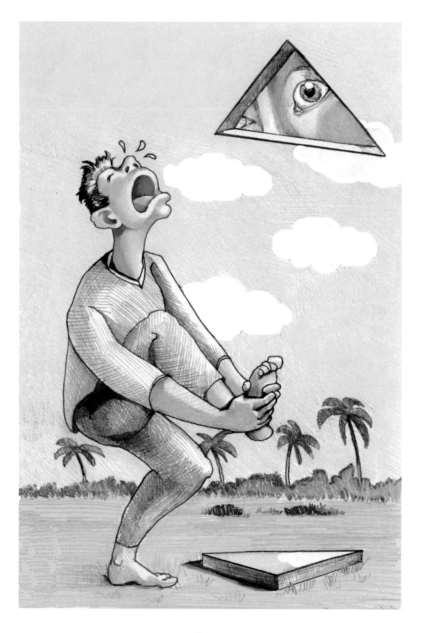

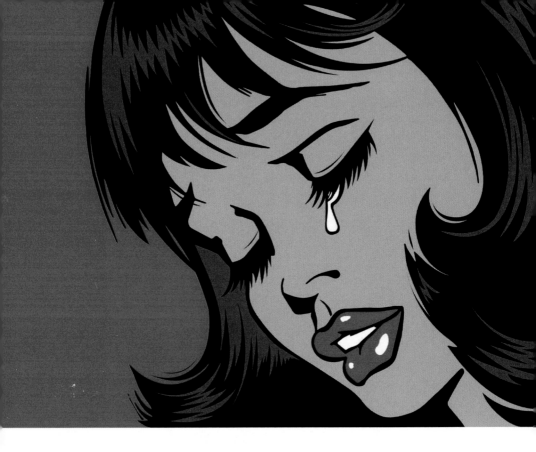

a. **<u>Acute pain</u>** is our brain telling us that there's an injury or illness we need to be aware of—**it's a warning.**

   i)   Annie breaks her ankle playing soccer.

   ii) She goes to see the doctor and gets an x-ray that shows her broken ankle.

   iii) Annie gets a cast and stays off her ankle for six weeks.

   iv) In six weeks, Annie's cast comes off.

   v)   **Her injury has healed and her pain is gone.**

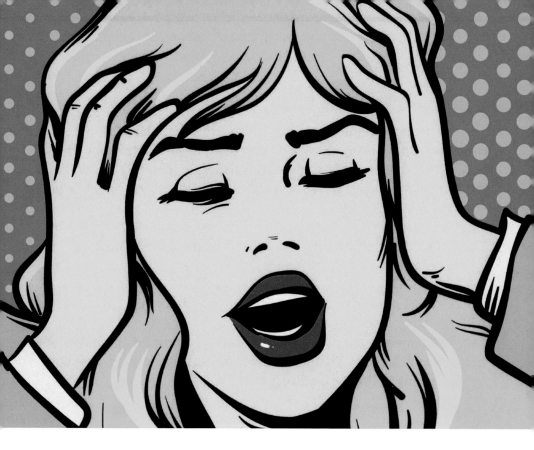

b. **Chronic pain** may or *may not* be our brain and body telling us there's an injury or illness. Chronic pain *stays* after the injury or illness has healed and **the pain no longer serves as a warning sign.**

  i)   Jenny breaks her ankle playing soccer.

  ii) She goes to see the doctor and also gets an x-ray that shows her broken ankle.

  iii) Jenny gets the same cast as Annie and stays off her ankle for six weeks.

  iv) After six weeks, Jenny's cast comes off.

  v)   **Her injury is healed, but she still feels pain.**

There is no more damage to either ankle—they both healed—but **Jenny is now experiencing chronic pain.** It comes in many different forms, and chronic pain is now recognized as a specific medical condition **related to an overactive nervous system.** The carpentry is fine, but the electrical system is off!

The first reaction of most doctors is to look at the ankle, because that is where Jenny experiences pain. *But,* that is not actually where the pain is—it is *occurring* in the brain. Even though it feels like there is pain in her ankle, **all pain is actually *processed* in the brain.** It's like a soldier with *phantom limb syndrome* insisting that his leg hurts even after it has been amputated. There's no physical leg there anymore, yet he feels pain in the limb. **That is because the part of the brain that controlled feeling in the leg is still active.**

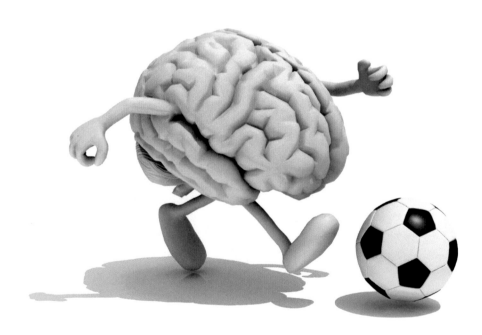

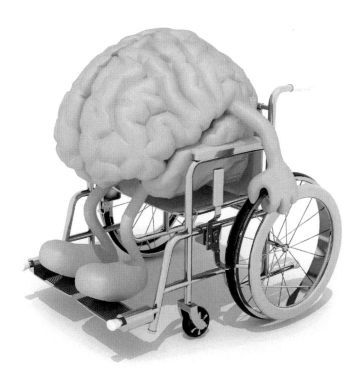

Chronic pain is real and can last for months or years. It is more difficult to diagnose and treat than acute pain because the actual sources of pain are more complex. Whenever we experience pain, **pain <u>receptors</u> are activated.** *They tell us we are in pain.* For most people, when the injury is gone the pain receptors deactivate. That's acute pain. *But,* with chronic pain, the pain receptors in the brain **stay activated**—past the healing of the original pain.

How do we start to solve this puzzle? Have you ever worked on a jigsaw puzzle? Some people start picking out all the edges to make the border. Others group pieces together based on color. You may even recognize certain details from the picture on the box, so you'll have a general idea where those pieces belong.

Just like every mind approaches puzzles differently, the same can be said for the approach to pain. There is no single right or wrong way to complete a puzzle. Similarly, our brains organize some pain as "chronic" instead of "acute." So, let's think of another way to solve the puzzle. *Easier said than done, we know.*

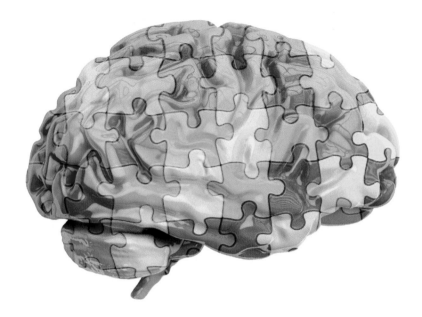

Maybe, instead of looking at the colors, you should try grouping by patterns or focus on the edges. Trying a new method means that you're already on the right path *(even if you may not know it yet).* Experiment with different ways to find what's right for you, because you won't know until it either works out or doesn't.

But sometimes things are misplaced. What if you lose the puzzle box and can't use it as a reference to see if you got it right? Sometimes you remember what the picture looked like; sometimes you can't.

People with chronic pain often feel lost and confused—like someone who has lost the top of their puzzle box. Their life may not have been perfect before *(whatever that means),* but with pain it's now more complicated than ever. In their time of need—when they *really* need help putting all their puzzle pieces back together—they can't find the box and can't remember where all the pieces are supposed to go. *What do you do with all of the pieces?*

The entire point of a puzzle is to fit the pieces back together in exactly the same way so that it looks just like the image on the box. It's a kind of *mosaic*. (If you don't know what a mosaic is, look it up on Google—they are really cool!) Every piece is arranged to make up a great and beautiful whole. Now, since we don't have our puzzle box picture and we've got all these pieces, why don't we expand our thinking? Instead of trying to force all the pieces back in the same old way that just isn't working, why don't we create a mosaic from them—our very own, new image? This is how problem-solving becomes more than just an activity, but an art form!

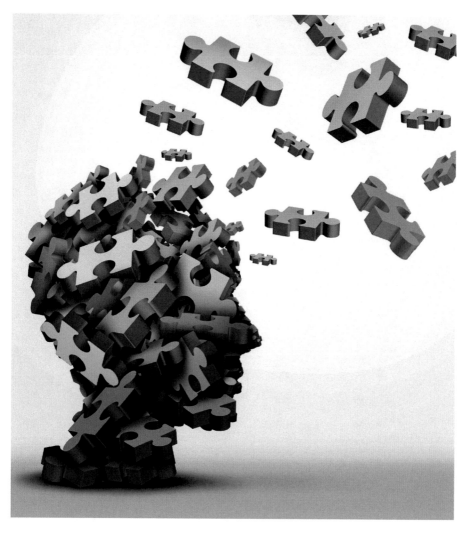

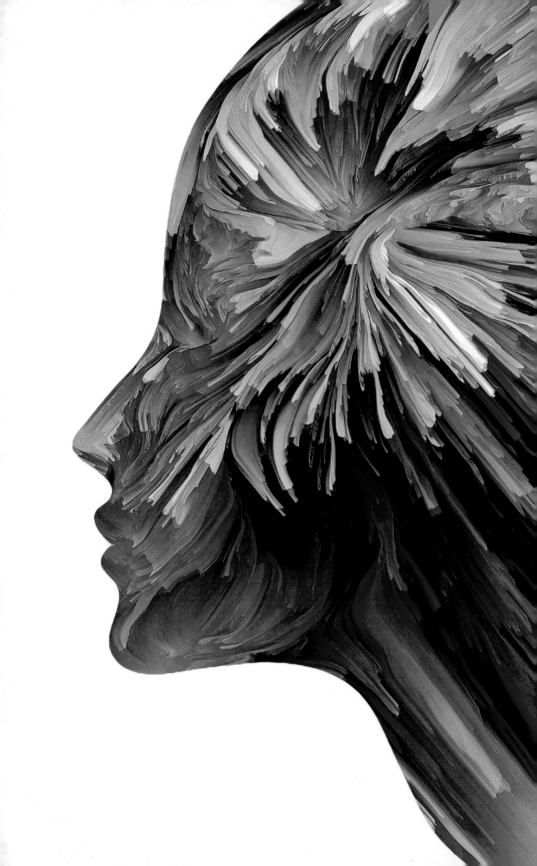

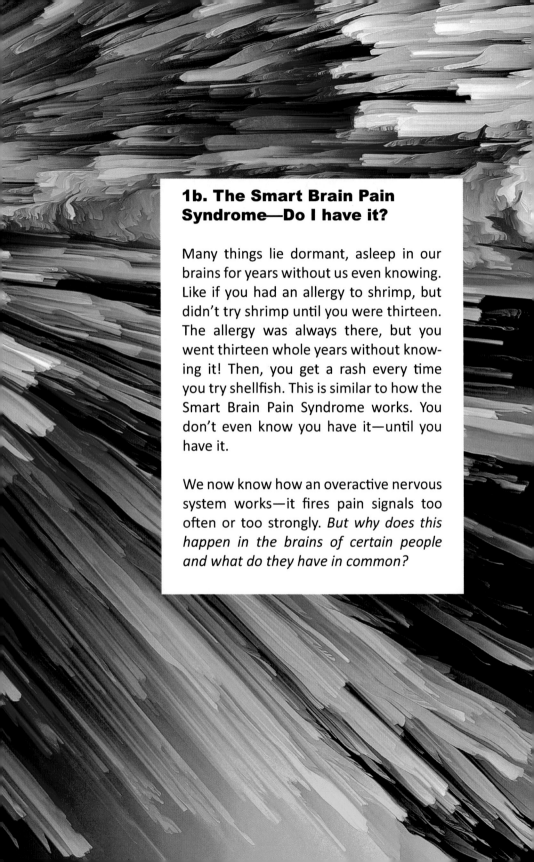

1b. The Smart Brain Pain Syndrome—Do I have it?

Many things lie dormant, asleep in our brains for years without us even knowing. Like if you had an allergy to shrimp, but didn't try shrimp until you were thirteen. The allergy was always there, but you went thirteen whole years without knowing it! Then, you get a rash every time you try shellfish. This is similar to how the Smart Brain Pain Syndrome works. You don't even know you have it—until you have it.

We now know how an overactive nervous system works—it fires pain signals too often or too strongly. *But why does this happen in the brains of certain people and what do they have in common?*

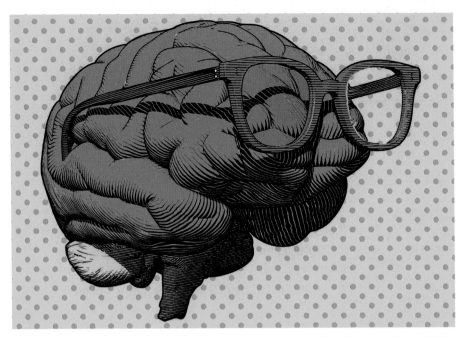

Bright ... Creative ... Sensitive ... Observant ... Perfectionist. Sound like you?

This is true of most people with persistent pain. These are all great qualities that make you special and unique, but they also make you susceptible to chronic pain! **Your brain learns so quickly and so intensely** that sometimes it becomes too aware, and **it gets stuck** *(which impacts your body)!* We'll get more into the nitty-gritty of this later, but it is important to understand that even though your smart brain is complicating things, **your smart brain is also your key to success.**

When people have ongoing pain, they are usually stressed. Your body can start to fall apart—*it's a lot to handle, day in and day out!* Have you ever ridden in an older car? The car is doing its best to get you where you want to go, but it's a long way! Even though the car is driving and working, over time it's not working as efficiently. It may start leaking oil or overheating more quickly, and **eventually, it may break down.** Maybe it won't break down completely but, while at the beginning of your trip you got 30 miles to the gallon, now you only get 10 miles per gallon. It'll cost you a lot more to go the same distance. This is the idea behind what's going on with your body. **The constant pain, tension, and stress are making it more difficult for you to get out of bed, go to**

school, and meet with friends. You may be able to keep going, but the strain can lead to everyday tasks taking a lot more out of you.

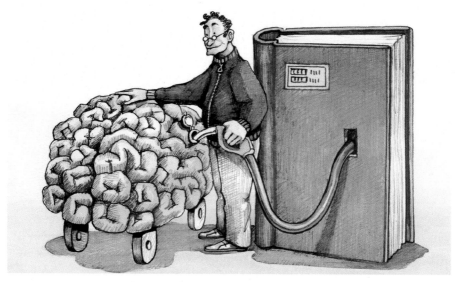

Let's look at stomachaches. *What happens when your stomach hurts?* You bend over and hold your tummy. If that ache doesn't go away, after a while that tension adds up. Gradually, the muscles on the outside of your belly tense up. **This causes more pain, and then more tension, and even more pain.** *Pain + tension --> more pain + more tension ...* it creates a kind of cycle.

The longer you are in pain, the more your brain is trained *("conditioned")* to be in that state. When we talk about "rewiring the brain," that refers to *deconditioning.* You can actually decondition your brain to your pain signals through **gradual exposure to things that make you feel good,** instead of focusing on negative feelings like pain and stress. You have to teach your brain that your body is okay, by showing it new and better ways to respond to those triggers: pain, stress, and fear. *How do we do that?*

We can't know if everyone reading this book *has* Smart Brain Pain Syndrome or not; it would be impossible to say. **But regardless of a label or diagnosis, the concepts and skills that we will talk about in this book are tools that you can use for the rest of your life.** So, why not keep reading and exploring all you can about the Smart Brain Pain Syndrome?

1c. Why haven't 14 doctors been able to diagnose my pain?

Doctors are traditionally taught a *"biomedical model"* of care. This means they look at a bunch of your symptoms and put them together to create a "differential diagnosis" *(meaning all the possible medical problems that this cluster of symptoms fits into).* Sometimes they do more tests to narrow down the actual diagnosis. This is a great method for diagnosing many health issues, but **chronic pain demands a very different approach** that some doctors don't understand.

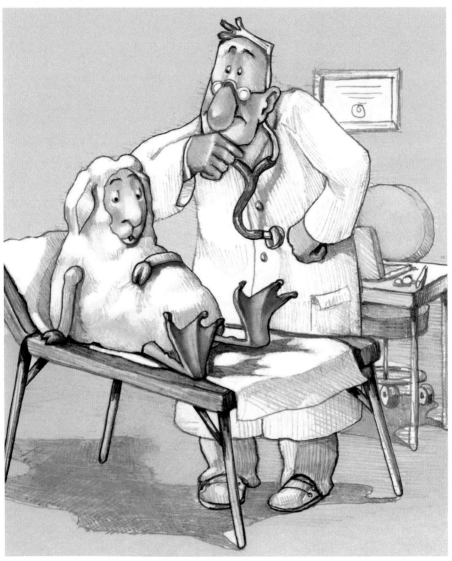

Diagnosing and treating chronic pain is like peeling back the many layers of an onion, because you have to look at the many factors influencing the whole you. We are not simple creatures; we have a lot going on. In addition to pain, we have bothersome siblings, peer pressure, parents telling us what to do—and what NOT to do. We have homework to complete and chores to be done. We have sports, hobbies, and activities that take our time and attention. *And don't even get us started on navigating friends and a social life!*

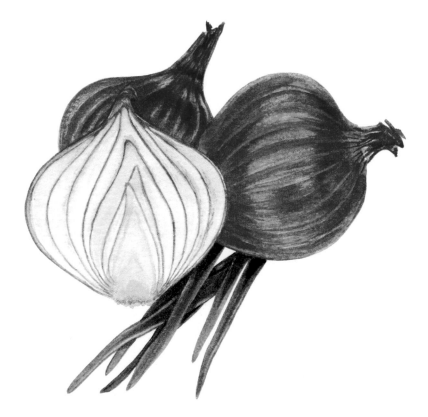

If the onion represents chronic pain, **every time you peel a layer it may expose another layer of issues that need to be addressed.** It's not quick or easy. It takes time, and even if some doctors have an understanding of chronic pain, most of them don't have the time to peel your onion and deal with all its different elements. It's very difficult for a doctor to truly understand you in the ten minutes they are actually with you face-to-face. This is not an excuse for them—it's an explanation for why you've seen many doctors who were unsuccessful in treating your pain.

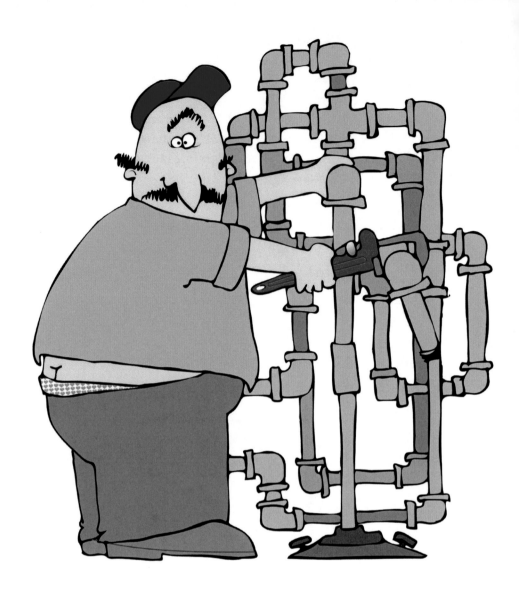

If you have stomach pain, you've probably seen at least one gastroen-terologist (the "plumbers").

If you have muscular or bone pain, you may have seen an orthopedic surgeon or two (the "carpenters").

Plumbers and carpenters are great at their crafts, but they may not be what you need. Instead of just looking at the pipes and woodwork, **we encourage you to explore your electrical circuits.**

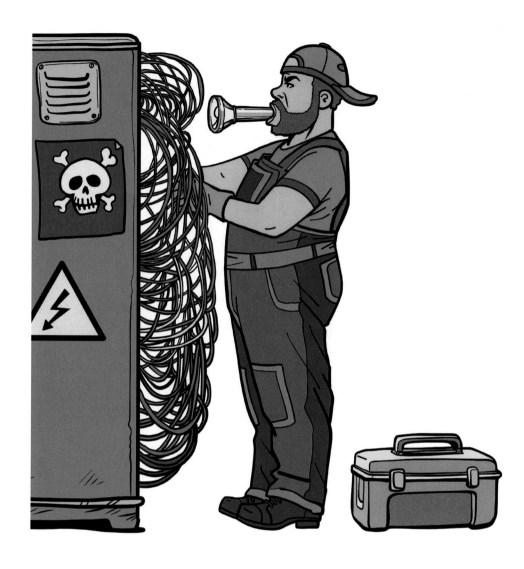

That's how we see our role—**the "electricians" of the body.** *What messages are traveling through your wires? What do your circuits look like?* There's more to a structure than just lumber and nails, just like **there is more to a body than organs and bones.**

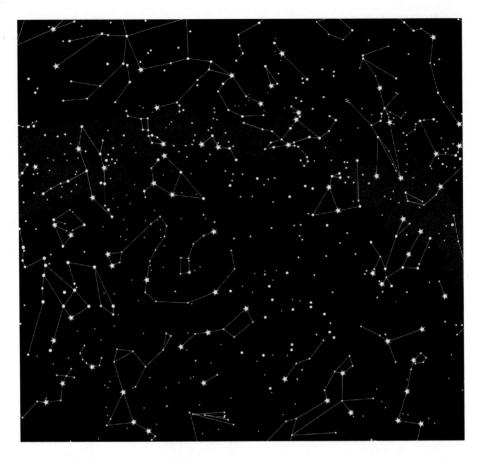

On average, most of our patients have seen 14 doctors before they see us (the record is 42). That's a lot of waiting rooms and assessment questionnaires, a ton of repeating your story and hoping each time will be different. *The answer has to be somewhere!*

We need to order additional tests for only one out of ten patients we see. **That means most of the answers have already been discovered; your history and tests just haven't been interpreted in a useful way.**

Looking at the big picture (using a holistic approach) is a special type of medicine that not all doctors can do. Diagnoses are like constellations—beautifully complex and haphazard at times. You can look at a massive sky full of seemingly random stars and slowly start to connect those dots.

Chronic pain can feel like a mystery novel. There is an unsolved problem, and you have many people following clues to explain the mystery. There are wrong turns and trips down rabbit holes. It takes a good detective, whether it be Sherlock Holmes, Nancy Drew, or Scooby Doo, to notice what is obvious, hidden, or hidden-in-plain-sight. The best detectives do not stop until the mystery is solved. **There is an answer out there—there always is. Sometimes that involves a combination of answers, but you will know when it's right.**

It will take time, but all problems have solutions—they're just not the easiest or most obvious. It is equally important to **recognize that not all solutions can or need to be explained at once.** This means that if it makes you feel good to sing proudly in the shower, or thoughtlessly finger-paint a "mess-terpiece," that's great! Keep that! Hold onto that action and feeling. Just because your neighbor may not appreciate you belting out tunes or your cousin disses your art, so what? *It makes you feel good.* **Explanations, to yourself or to others, don't matter.** When it's time for you or them or us to understand, we will.

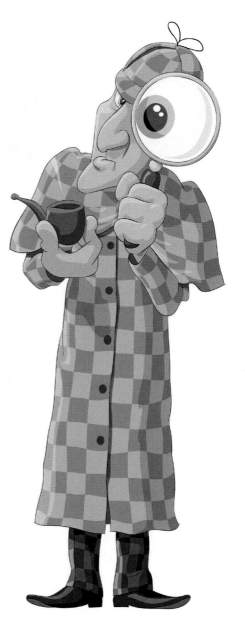

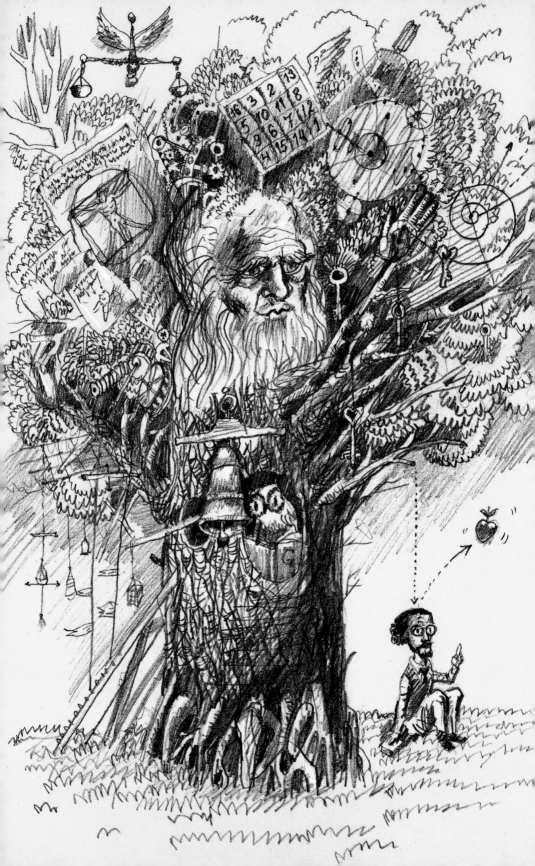

Look at how long it took to explain gravity. That is something that everyone knew about—if you have an apple in your hand and you let go, it falls—duh. But it wasn't until Sir Isaac Newton in the late 1600's that we really started to unpack the forces causing gravity. (Of course, not all explanations were correct off-the-bat, but they were building blocks!) And he did it while quarantined from the Great Plague!

It's interesting how Newton is often described as "discovering" gravity. He didn't "discover" it—humans knew about it long before he came around. What he did was try to *explain* it. And now we have the term "gravity" when we want to describe that constant pull.

It doesn't mean that gravity didn't exist before the term was created. The scientific explanation just hadn't joined our language yet. When you experience something, like the peace you may feel sitting under an oak tree or the energy you connect with as you dance, **you don't always have to label it in order to acknowledge its power. Creation of words and definitions don't change what things are, and neither will placing a label on your pain or experience.**

It is horrible to feel misunderstood. *How can something like gravity (or your pain) have gone unrecognized and unexplained for so long?* We don't have a great answer for that, and the answer, honestly, doesn't really matter. They are both palpable forces that affect everything around them. Geniuses like Galileo, Brahe, Kepler, Newton, Einstein, and others built off each other's ideas to develop our knowledge of "gravity."

There will also be many people with ideas that you will build upon and put your own spin on until you have the explanation that is right for you. Just like what eventually happened with gravity, you will solve your own mystery in time.

Chapter 2: The Brain

2a. Is the pain all in my head? Did I make it up?

No! Just because the pain is literally in our brain **does <u>not</u> mean that it is made up.**

Technically speaking, everyone's pain is "in their heads," since **that's where the pain receptors' messages from your stomach or legs are processed and memorized.** It's the electrical activity in our brains that tells us whether it's a feather or a rock that is brushing against skin on our arm or leg.

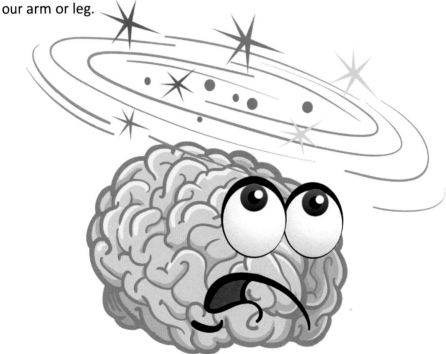

Just think about the difference between those two objects for a moment: a feather and a rock. There was no other description of what these things felt like. But **since we all have previous knowledge and experience** with a feather and a rock, we have learned what they feel like. Even though we don't have either touching our skin right now, we still can distinguish one sensation from the other.

When we experience other sensations *(like pain, pleasure, discomfort, tension, stress, relaxation, and many more),* our brains start to learn what causes each and what results follow. This process is not identical for everyone.

Think of your brain like a map—because it kind of is! It has lots of routes and tunnels through which electrical impulses run back and forth, sending us information about our experiences, creating our thoughts and emotions, and leaving the brain with our responses. And, **we know that the smarter our brain is, the more details we probably have on our map.**

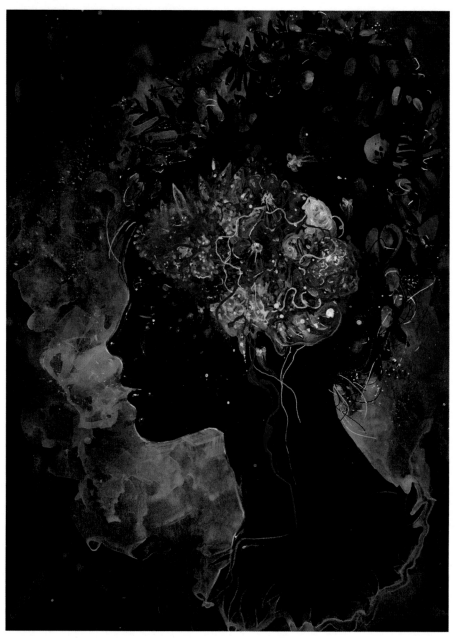

Keep imagining a map. For the sake of this exercise, let's focus on North America. Even though we have the ability to zoom in on details like the Golden Gate Bridge, we don't always need to think of specifics. It would take a lot of energy to constantly think about every detail we know. **Since our brains are so smart, they make shortcuts (filters) for us, to make room for new information.** *How nice, right?*

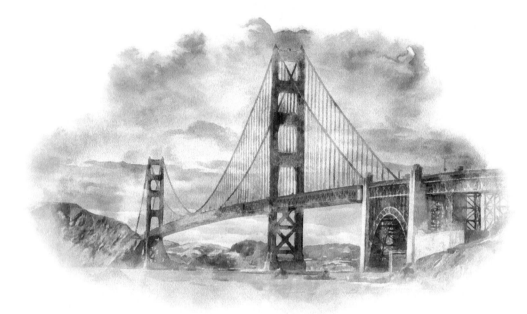

Since right now we're reading this book, we don't need to be thinking about the Golden Gate Bridge. So, let's zoom out.

Now, we may see the city of San Francisco, a cluster of buildings tucked tightly around the bay. Eh, that's still not necessary. Let's zoom out a little more.

Ah, California. We know the shape well. One more zoom out...

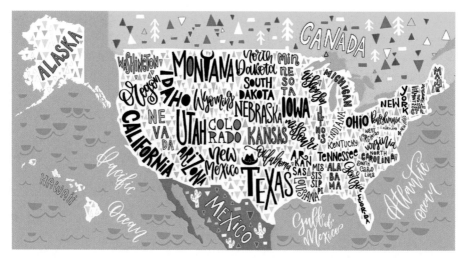

There it is—the United States of America! We see the smooth lines of the west coast against the Pacific. We follow the jagged edges down the east coast until Florida sticks its tongue out to separate the Gulf of Mexico and the Atlantic. We know the general shape, tucked in a sandwich between Canada and Mexico.

Now that we have zoomed out *(now that we are aware of more)* we are essentially more intelligent than if we were just able to know about or focus on the Golden Gate Bridge. We can see where Utah is—and Tennessee—all the way up to New Hampshire. We may know that even though Alaska and Hawaii are not close enough to be included in our "mind-map," they still exist—even though we may not be able to see them at this moment.

We know the general geography of the entire U.S.—we've learned it over the course of our lives. So, as we look at the country as a whole, we also have the ability to zoom back in on certain things we may need. Is someone talking about the deep-dish pizza in Chicago? Zoom in on Illinois to access all the information our brain has organized about that area. *Remember the cheese and grease running down your chin?* Phew, we were prepared for that topic.

And even though we may not know exactly where the Grand Canyon is, some of us may know it is in the lower left of our map. **We can sense the general direction because our brain has picked up on many hints over our lifetime**—that it is in a desert, and we know that the southwest tends to have the most deserts in the country. So, this knowledge is **based on an assumption, but it is also right** ... Is that a conclusion that our smart minds made without any concrete reason or previous knowledge that most of the Grand Canyon is in Arizona?

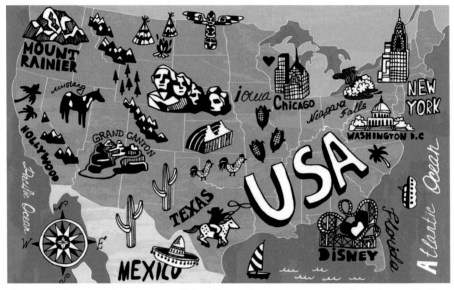

Once we know where everything is on the map, we can't *unknow* it. For example, can you forget about New York? Pretend there is no Texas?

It doesn't work like that. We already know too much about each of those places not to imagine them. Keep in mind, this does not mean that everything we "know" is always correct. *Hate to break it to you, but not all New Yorkers drink coffee and not all Texans wear cowboy boots!* But, until something corrects or *expands* our knowledge, we will continue to know what we know—and that's the best we can do.

The point of all this is not to brag about how much geography we know or how many states we have visited. This map of the U.S. *(or wherever you feel most comfortable imagining)* is an easy way to visualize our brains and how they process memories. Just as a map of the country can put us in different moods or trigger certain memories, so can pain.

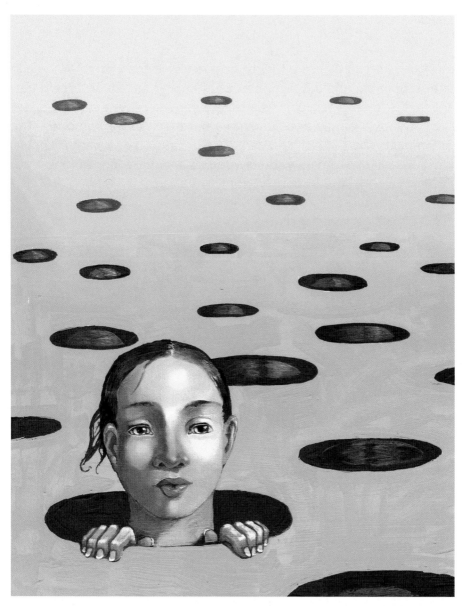

Even though our brains try to be our friends and look out for us, sometimes the shortcuts they create cause more trouble than good. It can oversimplify the route from coast to coast by saying, *"Keep going west until you reach the ocean."* Or, it may make our path home seem way too complicated by including nonessential details lining every road. **We will all get to where we need to go, but some brains make it more complicated than others.**

Most of us regularly use a GPS to help navigate the world. We type in our destination, and the computer usually gives us two or three different routes to take. Yes, each is a way to get where we need to go, but they are not the only directions *(and not always even the best)*. The GPS repeats the same thing every time because that's what it knows, while we can experiment with new routes and make innovations.

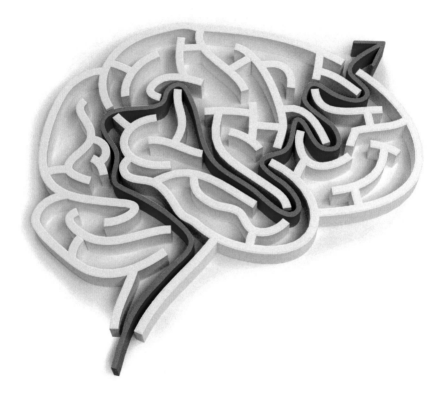

We recognize patterns based on our experiences and can make decisions on new, faster routes based on our prior knowledge. Even though the experiences of our life *(i.e. things that have happened to us or that we have learned)* may have taught us to make a left at the blue house or to stop next to the lemon tree, that doesn't mean that we can't explore new routes.

A lot of time our learning of pain is based on fear. The fear is that what we are doing (or have done) will cause harm to our bodies. So, our mind makes those same kinds of assumptions that it made about the location of the Grand Canyon earlier.

Think of taking a hike at the Grand Canyon and rolling an ankle. We remember the desert heat on our skin. We noticed a lizard scurrying by. We heard our mother yell. Remember when our brains already generalized the region earlier? Well, the same thing is happening inside our smart brains during this specific pain incident.

We rolled an ankle. We'll survive. But we know with utmost certainty that it is not an incident we want to repeat. So, we learn from it ... and the pain it caused (usually subconsciously).

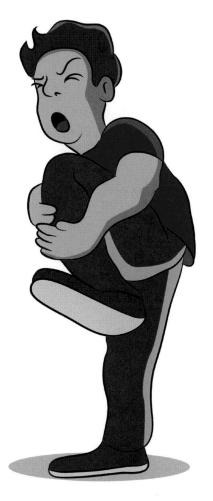

Think like a brain for a moment: what do we remember?

1. The heat: We were doing physical exercise. We were hot and sweaty. Maybe that is what caused me to fall. *Let's not do that again.*

2. The lizard: Small moving objects may distract us and prompt a misstep. *Stay away from chihuahuas because they might make me fall.*

3. Mother yelled: Mom is in distress when we are in pain. *Now when she sounds upset (even if it is just because she found a spider in the shower and has nothing to do with me), my brain makes me remember when she cried out on that hike.*

All of this happens automatically—these are the shortcuts that our brains take (also called associations). In reality, it wasn't the heat or the lizard that hurt your ankle. It wasn't even the fact that our Mom yelled, because we know that happened right *after* we fell.

So how did that simple experience change my brain?

- The simple truth is we may have stepped on a rock or worn the wrong shoes that day.

- It could have no relation whatsoever to any of the things that our minds noticed and used to create the shortcuts.

- Even though our brains are smart, they don't automatically *reason.*

- As a result, our brain may overgeneralize the entire experience and label Arizona as a "bad place" that we shouldn't return to because that's where we first hurt our ankle.

The next time we are in hot weather, the pain starts to warn us. If we see quick-moving objects, we feel fearful as they remind us of our tumble. People yelling causes us to think of our mother's horror, and we feel guilt.

But don't worry! Even though our smart brains may do this more than we want them to, that's okay. Just like we learn any other type of information that adds to our "mind-maps," we can also intentionally add or change routes.

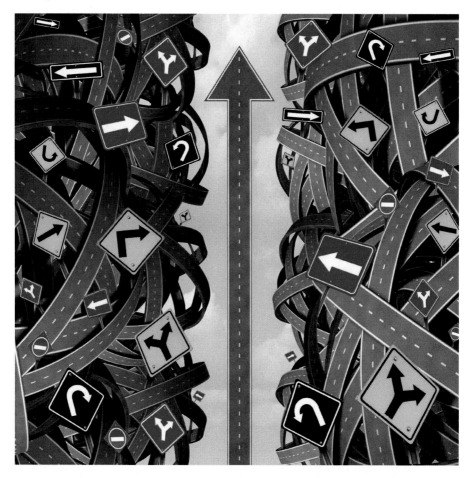

We can learn how to go down the same street, come up to the same intersection, but turn in a different direction. **We don't have to focus on or follow the path that reminds us of our pain,** because if we spend all day on that road, we can miss out on the more pleasurable journeys out there.

So, let's zoom in and out as we please. **Let's understand how to positively manipulate our smart brains into perceiving experiences the way we want.** *(This means teaching it what we want!)* And lastly, let's *enjoy* the process of rerouting the roads on our "mind-maps."

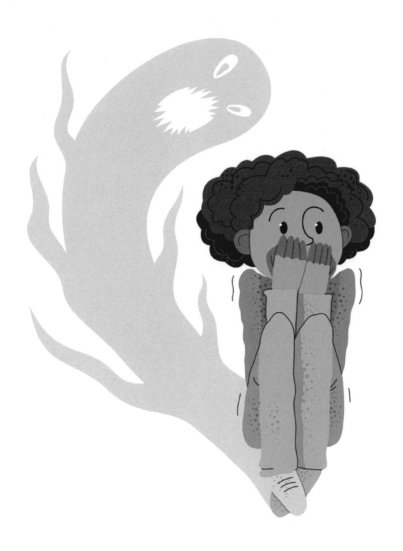

2b. How did my brain get stuck? How can I unstick it?

When the **autonomic nervous system** perceives danger, chemicals like adrenaline are released in the brain to help us survive. The "flight-fight-freeze" response is the mode that we go into to stay safe when we're put in a dangerous situation. For example, if we found ourselves face-to-face with a lion, some of us would run away, while others might pick up a weapon to fight. We are not here to say which is right *(and we hope you won't be put in this position anytime soon!),* but we do know that **this evolutionary reaction is designed to help protect us.**

Even when we're not in a life-or-death situation *(like coming face-to-face with a lion)* on a daily basis, there still can be subtle or **noticeable triggers for the same brain patterns.** This can occur when we hear a loud noise we weren't expecting or when our brother jumps out to scare us in a dark hallway. As a defense, our brains learn to react a certain way. **The smarter the brain and the more knowledge it has, the more connections can form to <u>confuse</u> the brain.** For some of us, instead of a lion being the trigger, it can be a critical teacher or an uncle who doesn't get it. There are many ways for this protection system to turn on, whether we want it to or not.

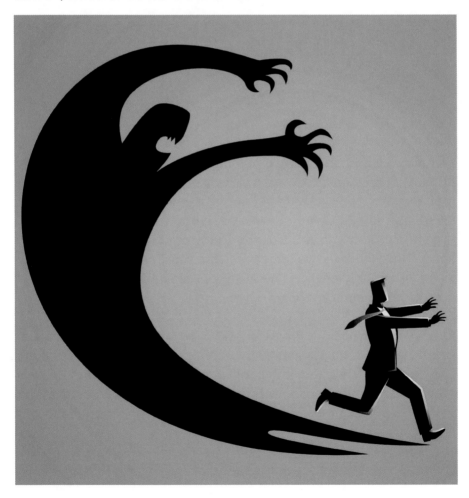

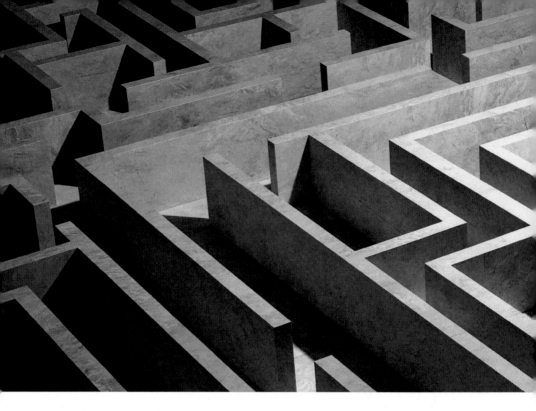

Each time your brain learns something, it maps out connections in the form of **neural loops. Your brain is like a maze that is constantly creating new paths and routes to get information back and forth.** Whether it's sounds, smells, sights, or sensations, our brain encodes this knowledge in our body—**that is how our body can learn from past experiences.** *Have you ever wondered why the smell of cinnamon can make you think of Christmas?* It is because your brain has made that connection, without you even trying!

Just as we learn positive things that stick in our brain (i.e. knowledge) to help us succeed, **the way we learn about pain also sticks in our brain.** Once we experience something, **our brain remembers it** and wants to keep our body prepared for it. **This can cause more pain messages that get stuck in the same sticky neural loop,** and thus ... we have chronic pain.

We know the problem: *what is the solution?* It's like reprograming a computer. Over time, everything has the tendency to get out of whack—yes, even your brand-new MacBook Pro! That means the system is out

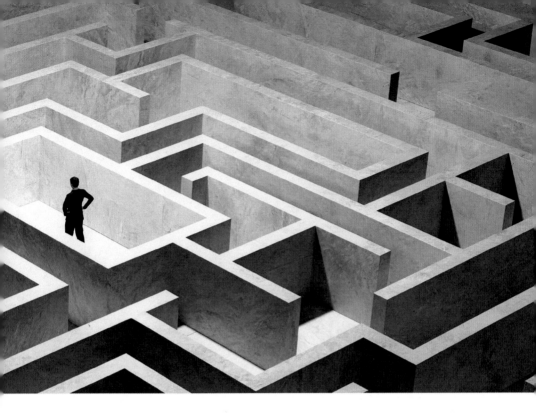

of balance and needs to be rebooted so the computer (and your body) can get back "in-whack." Obviously, we can't simply turn our brains off and on again like a machine, but the idea is the same!

The signaling system has gotten out of balance, which then leads to a number of other issues (like pain, sleep, fatigue, brain-fog, etc.). These difficulties lead to more complications, because when we are chronically stressed, in pain, or sleep deprived, **every cell in our bodies becomes stressed, in pain, and sleep deprived.** All the little energy generators in each cell *(aka our mitochondria)* get tired, too, so they don't work as well. That means they aren't generating energy, so then you start feeling fatigued.

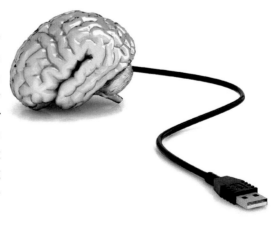

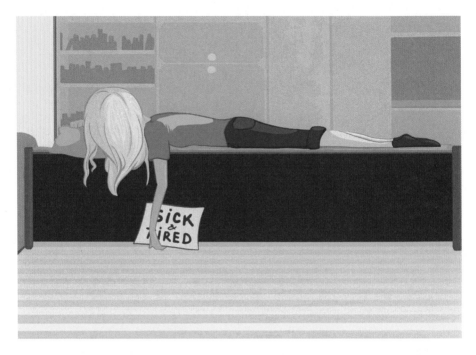

We humans, like machines, need energy to function. But, unlike machines, we have our own unique coding (our own natural bio-signature). *What does that even mean?* Well, in simple terms, it means that the "solution" for you is unique. Science has shown that a *Bio-Psycho-Social* model of care is needed to treat chronic pain. This means that neural-based mind and body strategies, plus social support *(feeling connected to others who understand),* are the tools needed to change the experience of pain. We like to call this creative healing. The most effective ways of changing those central pain circuits and reducing pain are not through medications (surprised?), *but through creative activities involving the mind and body.*

You never know when you're going to need a tool to help you heal. It's always a good idea to have a first-aid kit handy. Most first-aid kits include a Band-Aid, but a Band-Aid won't help if you banged your knee. That requires an ice pack. If you twist your ankle, that'll need a wrap bandage. Not every item can or should be used for everything – **that's why you need options to help you recover.**

Sometimes you may require additional assistance. That being said, you don't go to the hospital for every bump and bruise. Just like you have your Band-Aids, ice packs, and wrap bandages, **you can have your own tools to help you heal from pain.** If you expand your list to include more choices, you will have even more resources at your disposal. **That is creative healing—an alternative first-aid kit that not only treats your ailment, but over time can** *prevent* **it.**

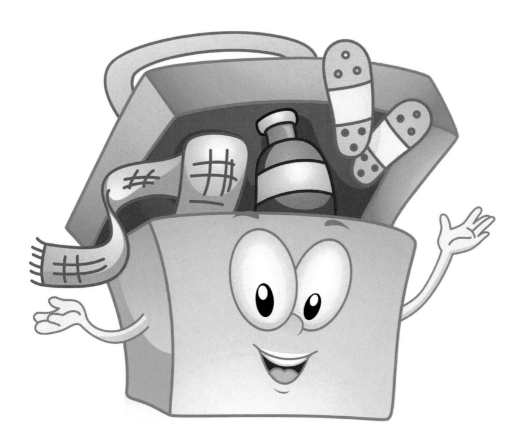

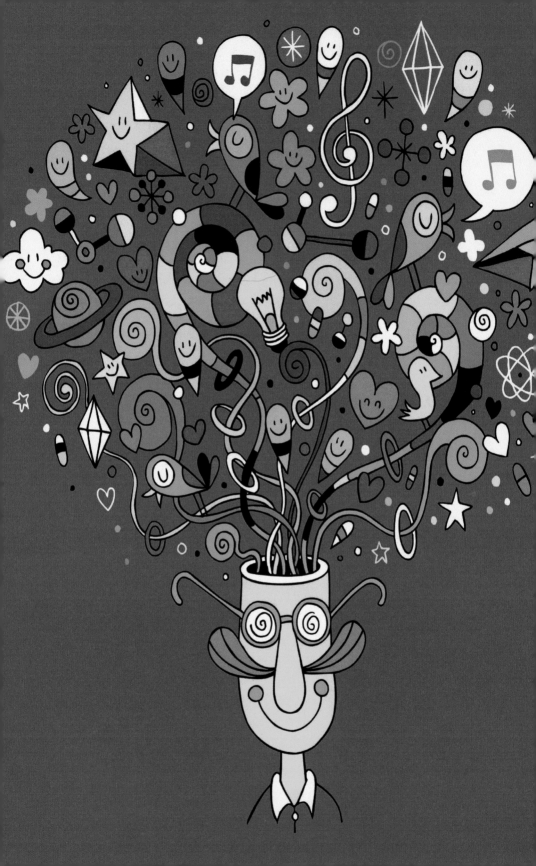

Creative healing first-aid kit: In addition to a Band-Aid, throw in a yoga class or two. Along with your cold pack, create a playlist of your favorite songs. Besides a wrap bandage, have a sketchpad ready to go. Sometimes you may feel the need to stretch or put pen to paper—other times you may just need to rock out to a good tune. **Knowing what helps you, having access to it, and participating in it can be the key to your healing process.**

Once you have your creative healing first-aid kit, you <u>will</u> learn how to "unstick" your smart brain and teach it to turn down the overactive pain receptors when they don't need to be working so hard.

2c. Is my pain harmful – or just hurtful?

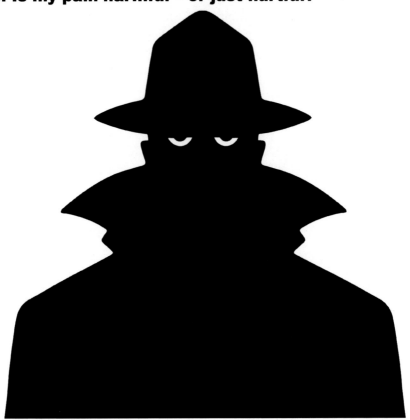

Pain is like having your worst enemy in the world know absolutely everything about you—**even things you may not have been aware of.** Even worse, **it can disguise itself, making you think or feel like your body is the enemy.** Don't worry, those are very common thoughts and feelings. But, when it is time for you to confront your enemy (your pain), **you will learn that your body is not the problem, but the solution. Your body (and your brain) will give you strength, show your progress, and help you accomplish your goals. Realizing that your body is your friend, with or without pain, is one key to rehabilitation.** A crucial step is learning the difference between *harmful* **pain** and *hurtful* **pain.** We admit neither sounds great—*who wants to be in pain?* But there is a difference which will become clearer once you learn what they mean.

Think back to when we discussed the difference between acute pain and chronic pain. It helps to think of acute pain as "harmful" and chronic pain as "hurtful."

Remember how acute pain alerts you to an injury or illness? It is your brain telling you, "This is causing damage," so **it forces you to give your body time to heal.** This is why we say acute pain is "harmful." **It is a protective response to reduce physical trauma.**

Chronic pain is more complicated. It is a *misinformed* version of pain. It is not necessary or needed to protect an injury, because there may not be any physical trauma there. **Again, this does not mean that the experience of pain is not real; it is real and we know it hurts.** But, since this kind of pain is not a reaction to "damage," there is really no need to give your body the same time to heal by lying in bed. There isn't anything "harmful" happening to your body that you need to address. So, that is why we refer to it as "hurtful." It doesn't diminish your pain, but there is a difference.

If you sprain your wrist in a tennis match but go right back to swinging the racket, you may be causing additional harm by straining the muscles when they are already weak. But if you sprained your wrist a year ago and it healed already, but it still hurts every time you swing the racket, **something else is going on.**

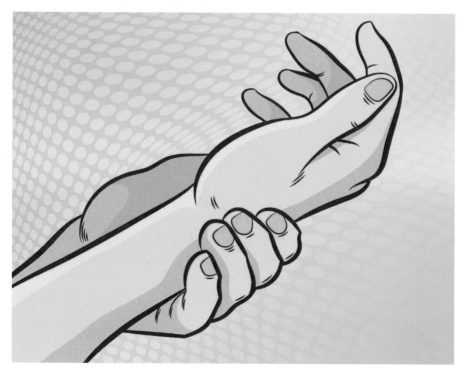

Once you stop fighting your body and start looking at its potential, **you will form that mind-body connection and reduce your pain. Your brain's reaction to pain is still trying to protect you, even if it doesn't need to. Your brain and body are doing the best they can.** It's like having a dog that's protective of you.

Take a moment to picture your favorite kind of canine. Imagine that dog in all its glory. It's your cuddle buddy when you're sad and your play pal when you want to have fun. That dog loves you so, so much. You are his or her source of everything—food, shelter, and affection. It doesn't want anything to happen to you, so it protects you and warns you of danger. **When it perceives a threat, it defends you.**

Not everything your pooch perceives as a threat to you is an actual threat. Not every stranger who walks through the door is someone who is going to harm you. So, whether it's the plumber coming over to unclog your toilet or a new friend you met at school, you show your dog that you are intentionally letting them in. You greet them at the door so the dog *sees* and *senses* that you are okay—this person is not a threat, so it can relax. Once the dog is calm, there is an opportunity for the pup to explore this new person. That's where the petting comes in and the oh-so-lovely belly rubs. *Who knows, there may even be a treat involved!* Over time, the dog **learns to trust your judgement, and it doesn't have to be "on-alert" anymore.** *It doesn't need to be in a constant state of fear or stress.*

Have you ever gone swimming in a pool with an anxious dog? Even though some canines enjoy water, most see your swimming as a sign of distress. They tend to run in circles around the pool and bark hysterically to alert someone that you need to be rescued. Swimming is a pleasurable experience for you, but the dog doesn't understand that because it doesn't associate the pool with pleasure because **it does not experience it that way.** The dog isn't trying to ruin your summer fun, it just **doesn't interpret it the same way.**

Think of your pain receptors as this dog. Dogs don't want to be worried — if you look at most of their undesirable behaviors, they **usually stem from being unsure of what exactly is a threat.** It may even come out as aggression like biting, or annoying behaviors such as barking, but that dog is doing its best. *And so are the pain receptors in your brain!* Just like how a dog may bark at the mailman while he's making a delivery, **your pain may be making similar exclamations,** alerting your skin to be extra tender to sensations. **Your dog can misread a situation, and so can your pain.** But, just like your dog can learn, **your pain receptors can learn, too.** *They don't have to be on constant guard, waiting for an intruder at your front door.*

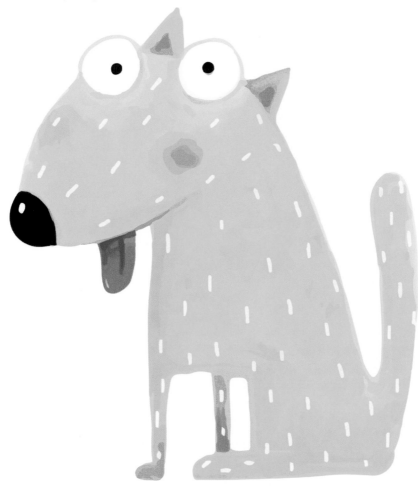

Just like your dog looks to you for guidance in new environments and unfamiliar situations, so does your pain. **It will respond based on your reaction to it.** If every time someone knocked at your door you ran under your covers, over time that would be the norm. *Same thing with the pain receptors in your brain!* If every time you hurt, you don't go to school and stay in bed, your brain learns to expect that every time you are in pain. Eventually, not only do you expect that, but your brain makes it happen, telling you to stay home.

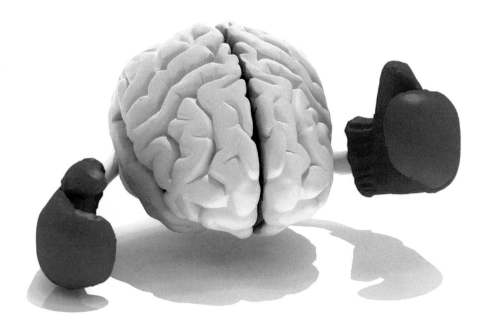

Obviously, there are plenty of times in life when it is good to stay in bed to recover, but remember we are talking about chronic, recurring pain here (once we have established the difference between what is harmful and hurtful for us).

But like we can't give up on our furry friends, we can't give up on ourselves. **We have to give ourselves the same unconditional love, compassion, and patience** that we give to our pets. When you find another chewed-up shoe or pee stain on the carpet and think you are at the end of your rope, you just take one look into your dog's big, all-telling eyes and know that it will be okay. *Do you know why that is? Why there is always so much hope and optimism in a dog's stare?* Because it is looking at you! Its eyes are reflecting what it sees in you. If we looked at ourselves the way our pets look at us, **we would have all the confidence and self-love we could ever need.**

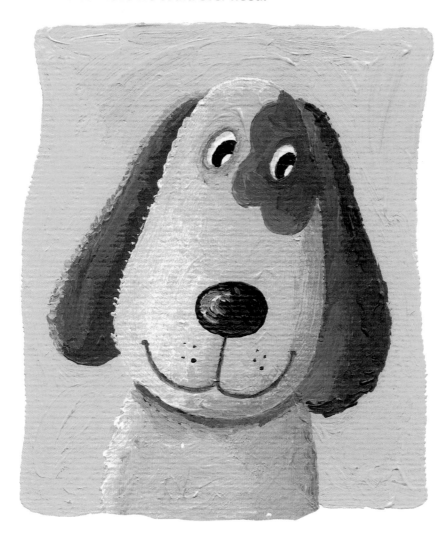

Chapter 3: Thoughts, Emotions, and Moods

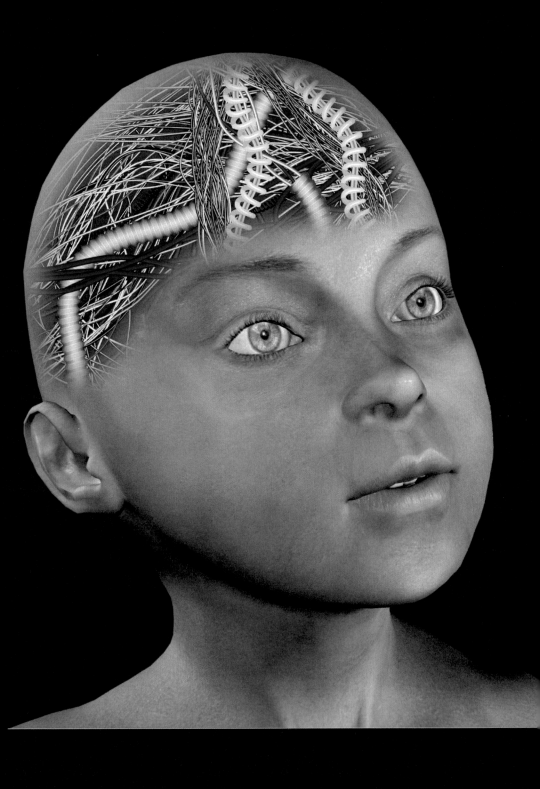

3a. How do I know when to think about my pain and when not to?

For most of our lives, when we are in pain we are told to "let it heal." *Don't pick at your scab.* *Keep your ankle elevated.* That's usually good advice. But here we are talking about when our smart brains are working harder than they have to, *interpreting pain when it is not always correct.* In this case, **function has to come first,** before the pain can go away. *Sounds backwards, we know!*

Have you ever been sitting outside at night, talking with a friend you really like? You're both cracking jokes and laughing—you're really engaged and happy during this chat. This discussion has your attention until it comes to an end (or maybe there is just a long pause). You may start to notice, *wow, it is reeeally cold out here ... why didn't I realize this before?* Odds are that the temperature outside didn't drastically drop in the seconds without dialogue. While you were talking and interacting, you were focused on the conversation. The cold was still there, but **you weren't paying as much attention to it.** And then you were.

Now, substitute the word "pain" for "cold." *See what we did there?*

53

Thanks to modern brain imaging, we have the tools to see what actually goes on upstairs. We can see the different areas in the brain that are part of pain signaling and study the pain "turn-off" system. *Pretty exciting, huh?* Well, it turns out it's a lot more complicated than just a message going up to the brain. We can now see **the path that it takes to get there.** As the message gets delivered it leaves an imprint, like a trail of breadcrumbs for the next time you have a similar experience. And remember when we were talking about how our brains make neural connections, but some brains get stuck in that pain loop for longer than is necessary? That comes back into play here.

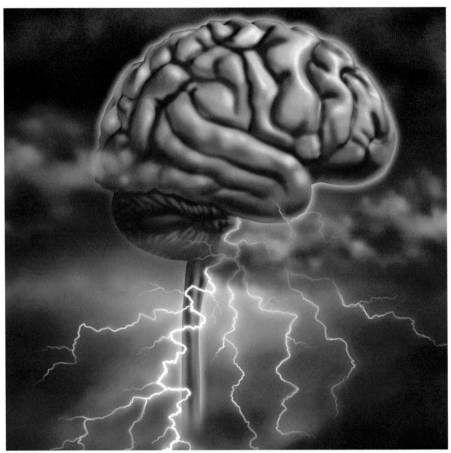

Imagine a busy highway going through a crowded downtown. **The highway is like the neural pathways that get developed over the course of your life.** They connect the different parts of your brain together (called the *connectome*). The highway is the route that the messages take going to and within your brain.

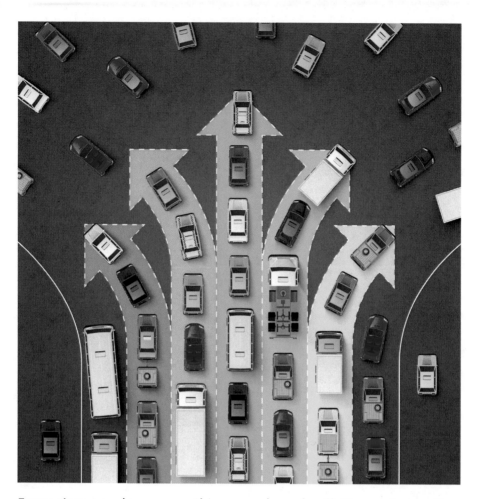

Every time you learn something, you branch off. You make another highway that your messages can veer off onto. And, over the course of your life, if you are learning *(which we all are constantly),* **then your brain is automatically forming new highways for your messages to travel through.** Some highways may put you directly where you need to go, while others take the scenic route—**but each highway is created for a reason.**

We even create highways in our brains for pain and, thinking back to that "sticky loop," our messages get busy and build up like traffic during rush hour. This is why you are feeling persistent pain—the cars on your pain pathway have been traveling up to the brain in masses. But, during your healing process, you can actually create a way to block the "bad traffic" and only allow the "good traffic" to drive through.

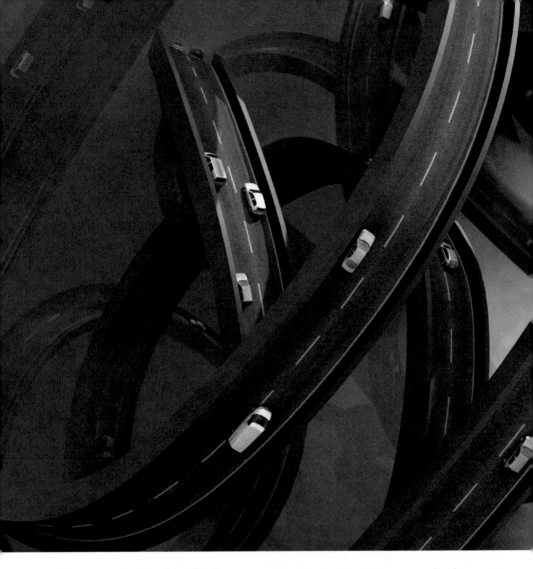

When we say "bad traffic," we are referring to the things we don't want to experience, like pain and stress. By "good traffic," we mean things that we do want to experience, like joy and relaxation. Throughout your healing process, you will figure out what kind of "good traffic" you want traveling on your highways. The more "good traffic" you can encourage to get out there on the road, the more it blocks the "bad traffic." **And, once your brain, mind, and body learn how the "good traffic" feels** racing effortlessly down the highway, **the more it remembers it** and saves space on those new highways for more "good traffic."

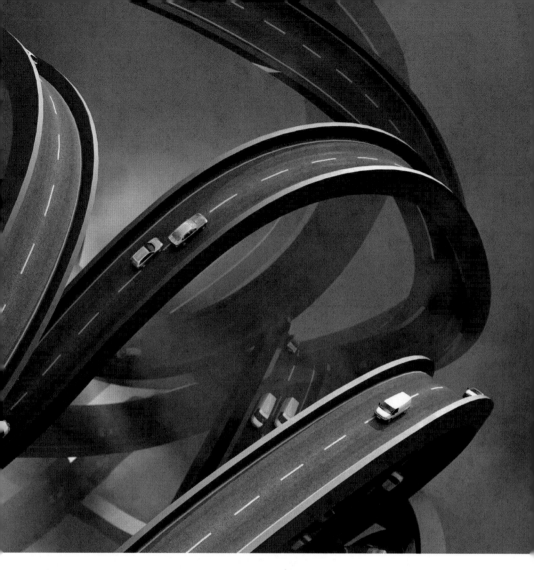

The more space on the highways available for the "bad traffic" messages to travel through, the more pain we are in. *So, how do we block the "bad traffic?"* Unfortunately, it is not as simple as closing a road, but there are ways to make the "good traffic" more prominent. In order to do this, what we want to really focus on is *attention.*

Even though this goes against everything we are trying to do here, think about your pain for a second. *Remember those unpleasant sensations? What do you notice?* You are probably feeling the pain, or maybe it is suddenly feeling *worse.* That's because **you are paying attention to it—you are letting the "bad traffic" out on the road.**

Now think of something you really enjoy doing. A common activity that most people do throughout the day is listen to music. *What happens while you are listening to music?* Are you following the rhythm as you tap your foot? Are you humming along to the melody you know by heart? Are you holding onto every lyric that speaks to you? Most importantly ... *how is your pain?* Believe it or not, when we are doing something we enjoy *(that grabs our attention),* it will **distract us from the pain and start the flow of "good traffic" rumbling through!** *Pretty cool, right?*

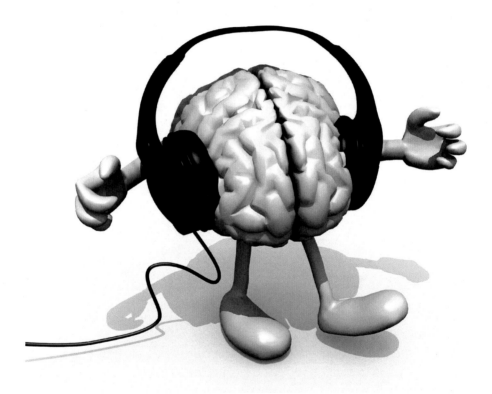

There is no "one-size-fits-all" formula for improving pain. Whether it be listening to music or cuddling with your cat, it's about doing different things that make you feel good and bring you relief and/or distraction ... with an emphasis on *doing*. **The <u>fundamental step to reduce your pain is doing things</u> and functioning again.**

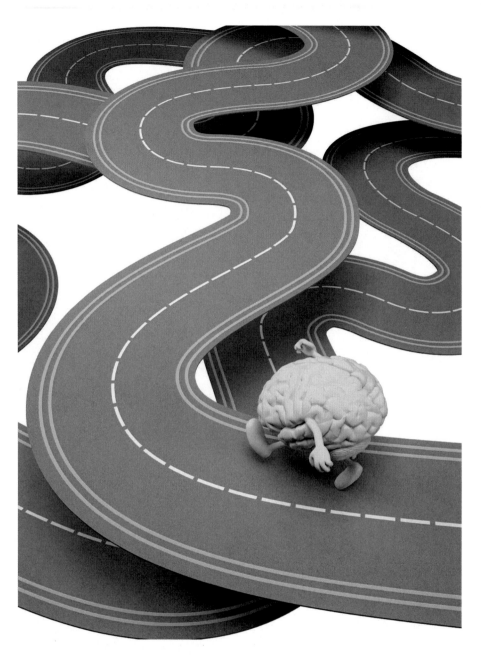

This is probably a hard thing to hear, but with chronic pain and our smart brain, the **disappearance of pain will be the last thing to happen.** What you have to do is actually **teach your brain that it's okay** to be in school. **Whatever challenge you're facing, show your brain that you can overcome it—because then your brain will relearn how to do these activities and will continue to send the "good traffic" through.**

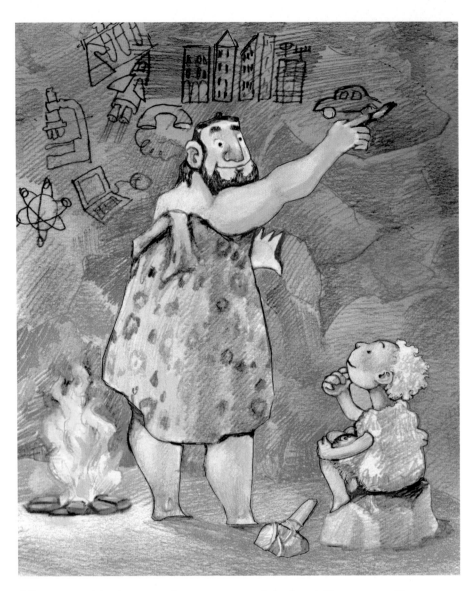

Of course, this does not happen overnight (and if anyone offers you a quick-fix solution, you should be skeptical!). Think back to every task or accomplishment you have ever completed. *Did that happen quickly?* Probably not. Even if it felt like an instant success, there were probably a series of experiences that happened beforehand that led up to it. *It's like learning the alphabet before learning to read and write, or going from crawling to walking to running.* **Day by day, you learned, experimented, and grew until you became skillful enough to move on to the next milestone.**

To answer the question in the title of this chapter ("How do I know when to think about my pain and when not to?"), the answer is pretty simple: **think about what you *want* to think about.** If you *want* to think about your pain, then okay, there's nothing we can do about that. But, at least now you know that will keep your "bad traffic" flowing, leading to more pain. On the other hand, **if you are sick of thinking about your pain and you are ready to think about the things you *want*—then what's stopping you?**

This does not mean that you can run a marathon and not have pain just because you're listening to your favorite jam in your earphones. Like anything, you should start slow and work your way up. It is about **gradually moving and *doing* safely**—this will not only help turn down your pain signals, but it will also **open a healthy dialogue between your body and brain.** Imagine them sending positive messages up and down your spinal cord, reassuring each other, "It's okay, this is fine ... in fact, this is *good!*" **Focus on the task at hand, not whether or not you are in pain.** Remember, even though pain may come and go, **where you put your attention is a choice.**

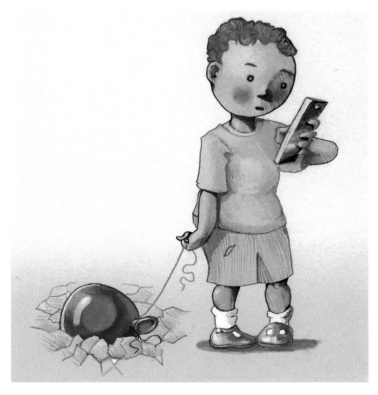

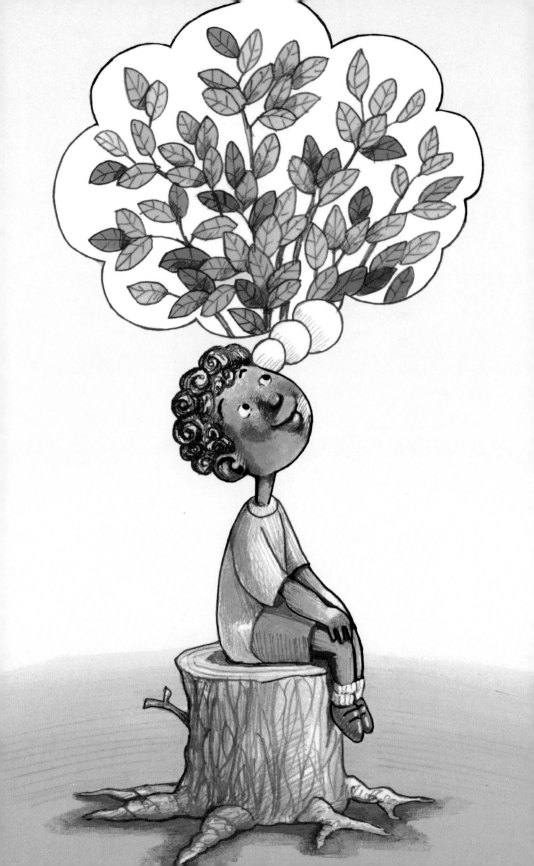

We use computers all the time nowadays. Whether you are on your phone or laptop, it may feel like your device is brilliant. Of course, it is, but computers have code that they have to stick to—it just repeats itself over and over again based on the circuits it was designed to follow. As humans, **we have the ability to *change* our circuits, even if they have been on repeat for a while.** We can make the *choice* to create a new highway or circuit on our motherboard. In a way, organic intelligence is a pretty special thing (maybe even more intelligent than computer "intelligence"), because it gives us the capability to **learn and grow.**

So, the next time you are in pain, give this a shot. *What do you have to lose?* Call up a friend, turn on your favorite TV show, or walk outside to smell the roses. Remember, **think about whatever you want to think about.**

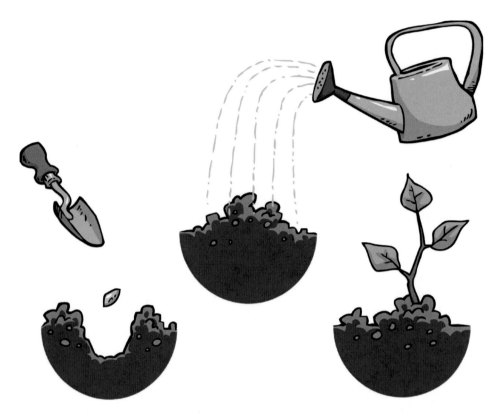

3b. How can pain affect my thoughts, emotions, and moods?

When a seed like pain is planted, *it grows.* You may not intentionally water it, but it still sprouts and the vines wrap around you like a weed with no mercy. You may try to block out the light—plants can't grow without sunlight, right? *So, I just won't leave the house today; I'll stay in my room with the windows closed.* Plants can't grow without soil, right? *I will make sure I remove any excess so there's nothing for the roots to hold; maybe I won't go to baseball practice today ...* and so on it goes. **Each decision you make, thinking you will prevent the pain from growing, actually makes it stronger**—until one day, it may be hard for you to even see the sunshine or feel the earth under your own two feet. **Pain, like any weed, can take over everything.**

Let's pivot for a moment and talk about languages. Even though all languages are beautiful and important, for the sake of simplicity we will use some specific examples. First, suppose you grew up speaking English, but then you started taking Spanish classes. Since English is your first language, almost all of your initial words will be in English. As you learn the basics of the Spanish vocabulary, your brain starts to translate certain words in your memory and your own vocabulary. So, when you hear the word *"hola,"* your brain turns it into "hello." That conversion happens over and over again with many words, until one day your brain doesn't have to actively work at it like a math equation. One day you will hear a word like *"hola"* and just naturally know what it means.

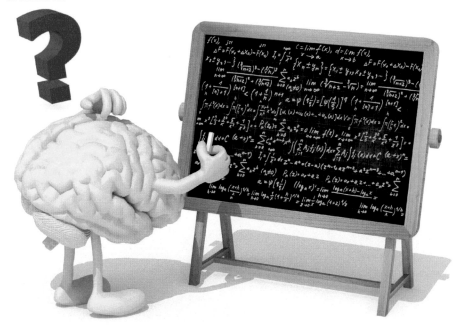

Believe it or not, **our bodies and brains speak different languages.** Since they are both part of you, **you may assume that they automatically understand each other, but they may not.** Your brain may be communicating in English, but your body is fluent in Mixteco or Tuyuca. These may be languages you've never heard of before, but that's the point. And honestly, **the actual language that your body "speaks" doesn't really matter—as long as you are open to learning how to understand it.** Because the actual letters and words don't really matter in this kind of communication—it is all about translation (which may not have any articulate alphabet at all).

Maybe your body's term for "happy" is the release of serotonin, or its way of expressing the word "comfort" is by relaxing all of your muscles. And, just like it has a way of translating positive things, it also shows you how it interprets phrases like "fear" or "pain" because it tenses up. **Recognizing your own body's language,** which does not include actual "words," **is how you can begin to translate it in your brain.** It's hard work learning this new language, but over time, understanding and communicating with your body can be as automatic as knowing the word *"hola"* means "hello."

The difference between *gliding* through this learning process and *stumbling* through is learning on your terms. It is one thing to be in an air-conditioned classroom with a pocket dictionary nearby, sitting next to your best friend as your teacher explains the information. It would be a completely different situation if you were dropped off in the indigenous regions of Oaxaca and Puebla in Mexico, where Mixteco is spoken, or if you found yourself wandering through a village in the Amazon where they only understood Tuyuca. That could be a little uncomfortable for a while. Just like you are probably not fluent in either of these languages, if you are not effortlessly communicating with your body and its pain, **it may be stressful to have these messages of unidentifiable information coming at you day-in and day-out.** That can lead to not-so-pleasant thoughts, emotions, and moods.

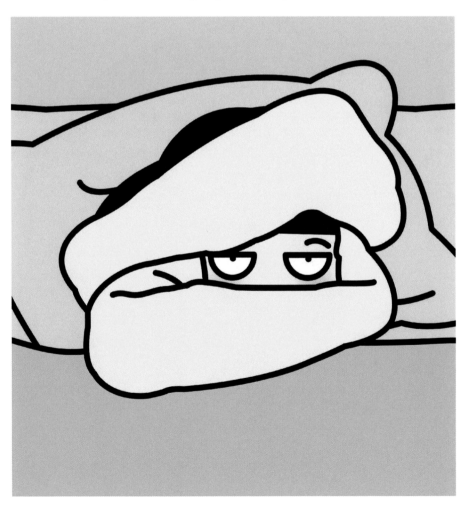

These three terms may seem interchangeable, but they're not.

> 1. Think of *thoughts* as something concrete that happen suddenly and consciously.

> 2. *Emotions* are something that we can feel unconsciously, without the ability to really visualize them.

> 3. *Moods* are triggered by thoughts, emotions, and more, but they may not be as clear-cut.

Have you ever found yourself in a bad mood and unable to identify why? Although these three experiences are different, they are not separate. They all influence each other and intertwine.

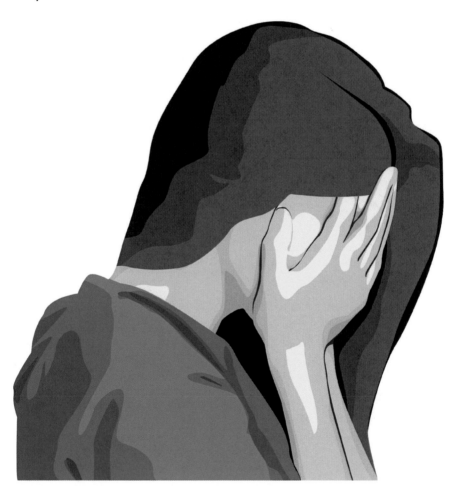

If you are in pain...

Your first thought may be: **"Oh no! This means I can't go to the mall today with my friends."**

Then, because of that thought, your emotions could be: **sadness or disappointment.** Those thoughts can lead to a mood like: **feeling gloomy.**

See what we're getting at here?

Resentment. **Sadness.** Anger. Frustration. Pity. **Desperation.** Unhappiness. **Shame.** Fury. Isolation. Confusion. Rage. Craziness. Indifference. Bad. Alone. Frantic. Explosive. Uncontrollable. **Wrong.** Intense. Unfortunate. Severe. Damaged. Guilty. **Worthless.** Sorry. Unacceptable. Fear. Worry. Miserable. Destructive. Negative. Vicious. Disaster. Terror. Nervous. **Panic ...**

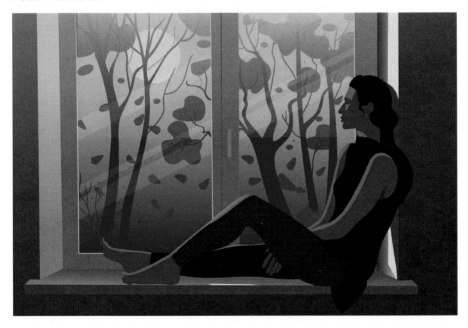

These are all common descriptions of what may be going on inside of your mind when you are in pain. That is normal. *What is something that all of these have in common?* They put you in **more distress because that is how this cycle works.** Just as pain can affect your thoughts, emotions, and mood ... **your thoughts, emotions, and mood can affect your pain.**

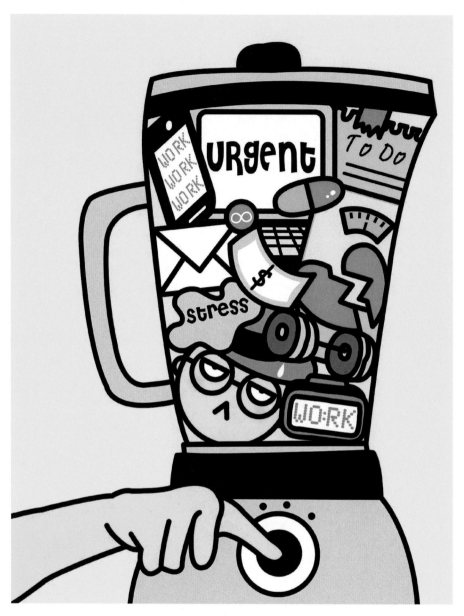

3c. How do my thoughts, emotions, and moods together affect my pain?

Fear is a major factor that impacts our pain through our thoughts, emotions, and moods. Those are the parts of our self-talk that fear lives off of. **Fear is our inner dialogue telling us that our worst nightmares are going to come true if we do or don't do something.**

If your fear tells you: "I may get a stomachache if I go to school today." Then, you may say: "I'm not going to school today."

Every time you fret, "If I get a stomachache, my teacher won't let me leave to use the bathroom," or "The school bathrooms are terrible and there's no privacy," **your body is releasing a stress response chemical called adrenalin.** That is what keeps our pain circuits going.

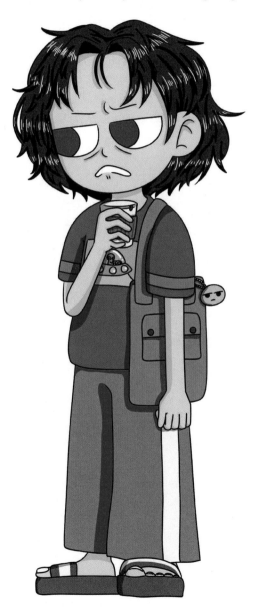

And even if you do go to school with that belief still in your mind, your sticky brain will hold onto that memory of your stomach pain that you had before and play it back for your brain—**reminding it to activate the pain circuits,** *even if they weren't on to begin with.* Remember, our smart brains take it upon themselves to protect us from what they perceive to be harmful by holding onto pain to remind us to avoid a situation, even if it didn't cause it. **Now, the fact that you are worried about being in pain can be what puts you in more pain!**

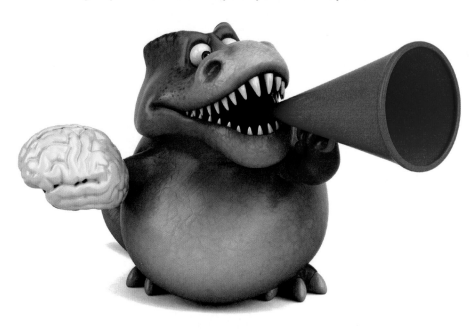

When we are anxious, we revert back to what is called our "reptilian brain." *(Yes, even humans have a **reptilian brain**.)*

Think back to the pictures in your science class on the evolution of monkeys turning into humans over time. The original monkey's forehead was pretty flat. But as the front brain grew with features like executive functioning and higher control functioning, the forehead extended to make room for our newly shaped organ.

This gave us the ability to pay attention and plan. **Our brains were able to create new neural circuits, making us more complicated and advanced.** But when we are put in certain situations that appear to be dangerous, our reptilian brain kicks into gear and we go back to the automatic survival thought process of our earlier ancestors (even if it is purely based on fearful thoughts, emotions, and moods).

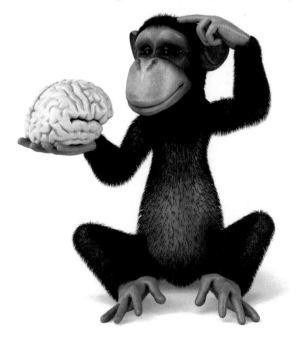

That is why **we don't want to live in our reptilian brains.** We can do this by strengthening the front brain with our evolved and intentional thought process.

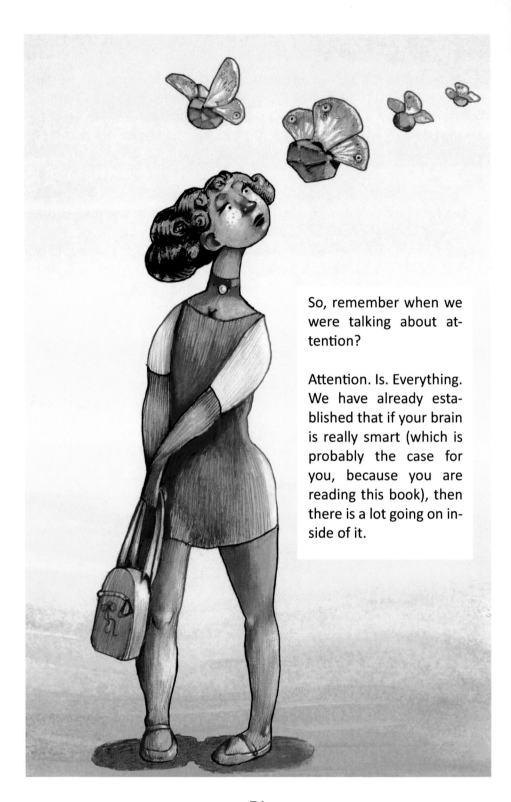

So, remember when we were talking about attention?

Attention. Is. Everything. We have already established that if your brain is really smart (which is probably the case for you, because you are reading this book), then there is a lot going on inside of it.

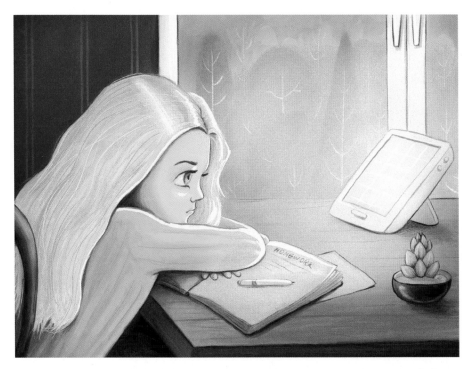

The act of **multitasking** *(doing multiple things fully and successfully at the exact same time)* **is not actually possible in the human brain**—at least not in the way we believe. Think about when our parents tell us to turn off the TV or put the cell phone away while doing our homework. We may respond with an exclamation like, "I can do my homework while I (insert activity of choice here)!" Even though some of us can *think* that we're multitasking, **it is actually our smart brains switching back and forth between tasks so quickly that it seems like we're doing them at the same time.** That doesn't mean we can't complete our homework while having the TV on or texting with a friend, *but* we're sorry to say that you are not "multitasking" in the way that you think you are. **Our brains can really only pay full attention to one task at a time, so it's actually rapidly switching back and forth:** TV --> algebra --> TV --> algebra --> TV --> TV --> TV --> algebra. We just don't notice because it happens so quickly!

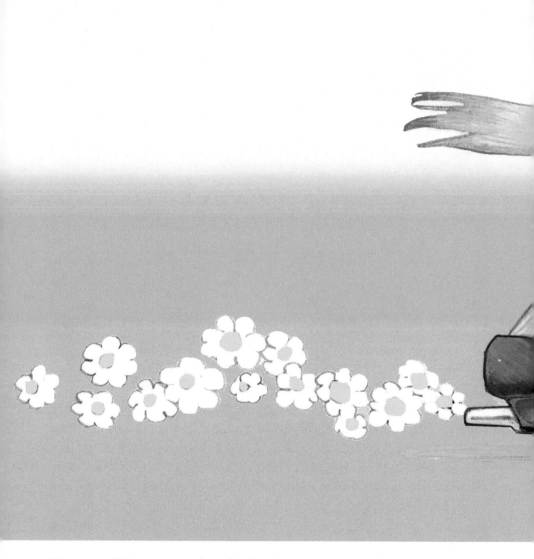

We can still be *aware* of multiple things at once. A lot of people can drive a car with the radio on or talk on the phone while walking. But *awareness* and *attention* are separate—yet often parallel—things. Speaking of walking, have you ever started from "Point A" with the goal of arriving at "Point B?" Maybe you walk one block and see a shirt in a store window that caught your eye—*oh my gosh, I need to try that on. Detour! Okay, they didn't have my size … back to traveling to "Point B."* And then you walk past a convenience store and notice how thirsty you are. *I'm just going to run in and grab a water …* Another detour!

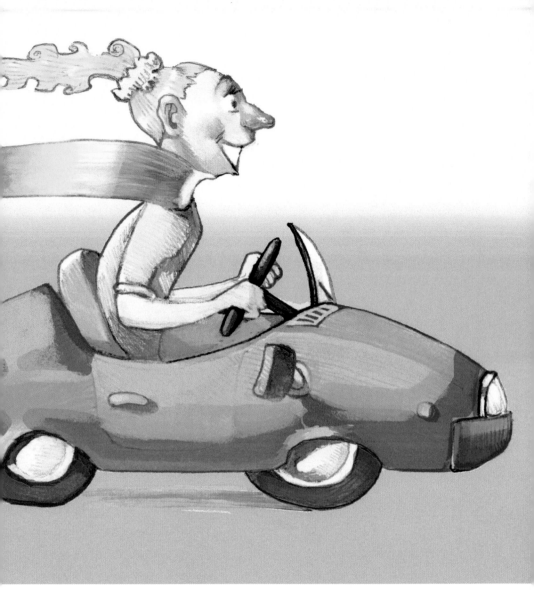

There is nothing wrong with detours, breaks, or a good-ol'-fashioned change of plans, because eventually you will arrive at your "Point B." But the point of this little detour is that our smart brains are like a popcorn machine with lots of thoughts popping around and changing where our attention lies. **When we notice that and make the choice to pay attention to something enjoyable (i.e. creative healing) instead of something unpleasant (i.e. pain), we have the power to reduce our suffering—by sending positive, *intentional* messages back and forth between our brains and our bodies.**

Chapter 4: Healing

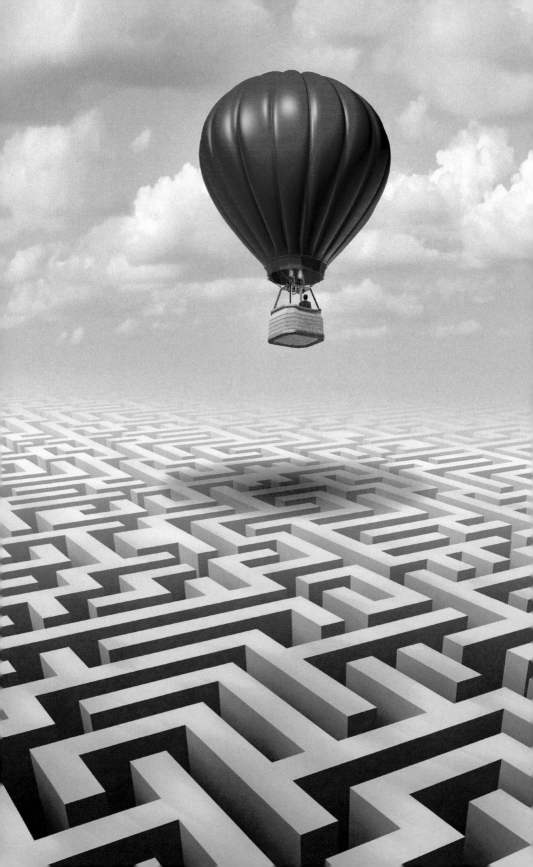

4a. My creative brain—it's both the problem and the solution?

Sometimes it can feel like you're stuck. Other times it seems like you have nowhere to go. *How does someone just restart their life out of the blue?* Like ancient explorers embarking on grand expeditions to faraway unknown lands, **you have the ability to create your goal *and* your route to get there.**

You don't even really need a "goal" to start a process or journey, because maybe your "goal" hasn't been discovered yet. Maybe there isn't even a map, since it is uncharted territory after all *(like your pain management so far)*. Perhaps all you need is a direction to start. The destination will be found when it's time, and the map can be created along the way. When you're paving your new path forward into an untouched land, it can be scary and intimidating *(like rewiring your brain's neural pain circuits),* but that is how villages are built into towns, which grow into cities—and greatness is established.

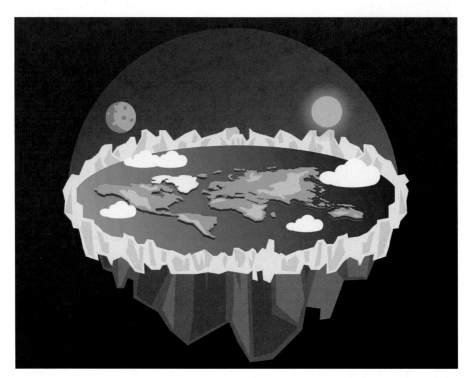

Some explorers had ideas about what they thought Earth was like—flat enough to fall off the edge! And it may feel like every once in a while, *you may fall off the edge*—but hold on—there are lots of ways to feel confident that the Earth is beneath you.

Again, you don't need to know the destination before you begin your journey. In fact, some of the best destinations are discovered through unplanned ventures. All you really need to know is that the ground you are walking on will support your weight as long **as you keep moving forward.**

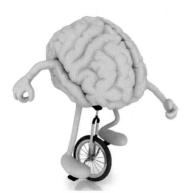

Some paths lead to dead ends—they just do. Some cliffs are impossible to climb and some rivers are too wide to swim across. But there are other routes—you just have to find them *(maybe even make them yourself!)*. **The paths that you will take to rewire your brain will be created in the same way.**

Once you have your route and you are familiar with the path, it takes the fear out of the equation. When you have a way out of pain, even if you have a relapse of pain again, you already know how to get through it. Since you created your healing path, it will be easier to navigate—and you don't have to be afraid of the unknown, because it is known to you. **Fear is the biggest obstacle in this process,** and once you remove that from the equation, you will feel more in control of your journey—*because you will be in control.*

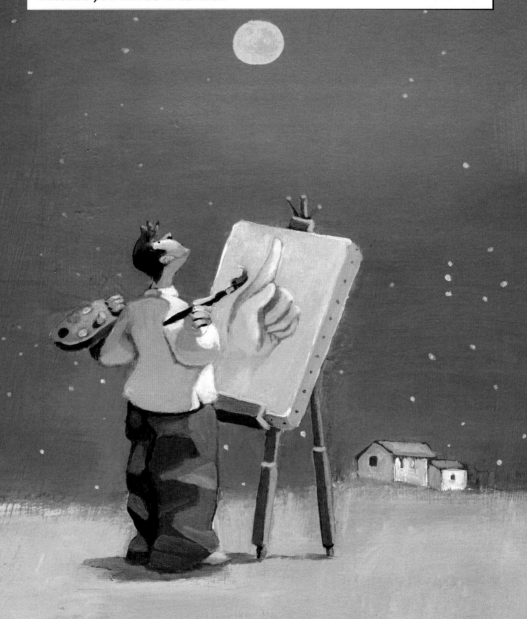

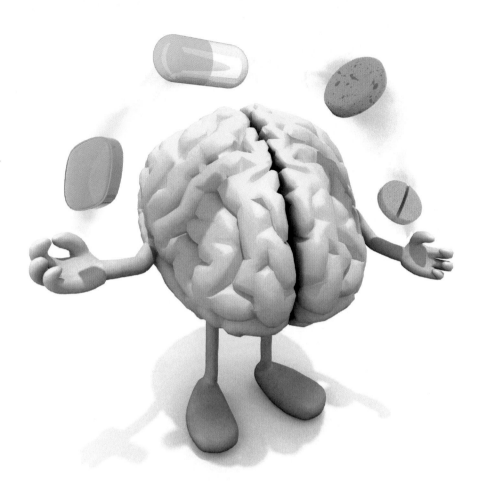

4b. Creative healing? How can it help with my pain?

Chronic pain is a neurological condition that occurs primarily in the brain *(with extensions to different parts of the body).* But—the "traditional" model, mostly medications and procedures, that most medical doctors are taught to use **does not** work for young people with this problem. Research has shown the most effective ways of changing these central pain circuits and reducing pain are <u>not</u> only with medications, but with **creative activities involving the mind and body.**

With this creative healing approach, **you can learn how to "unstick" your smart brain** and **teach it to turn down the overactive pain receptors** when they don't need to be working so hard. You have pain because of your high-functioning mind and intelligence. So, by **strengthening the mind/body connection** with creative healing activities, **your brain will teach itself new ways to experience information.**

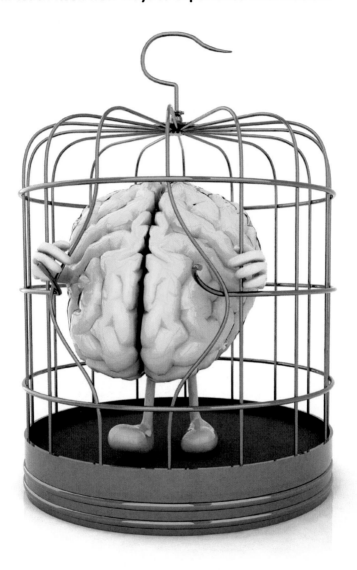

Creative healing is something that you are already doing, *whether you know it yet or not.* Everyone copes in different ways. Something to remember is that there is no "wrong" way to heal. Every decision that you've made thus far has gotten you here today, so you should be proud of that. That being said, there is always room for growth, so it is great that you are open to learning more.

THE TOOL KIT

Life is all about options. If you look at who society decides is "successful," it isn't solely about the money they have—**it's about the options available to them because of their adaptable resources.**

Resources can include people and relationships. They can consist of skills or materials. They can even be comprised of your own intelligence. And that's exactly what creative healing is—**using your own resources to help with your health.** *Let's start by jotting down some of the resources you already have access to:*

    1.   <u>Example: A playlist of my favorite songs</u>
    2.   _____
    3.   _____

There are some more! Hmmm ...

Whom do you have in your support system?

    4.   _____
    5.   _____
    6.   _____

What are your strengths? What skills do you have?

    7.   _____
    8.   _____

What are you interested in?

    9.   _____
    10.   _____

Okay, great. Your list is really coming along!

Next, let's build your toolkit! Here is a list of options to get you started ....

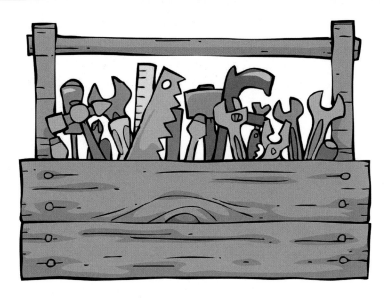

My Toolkit For Getting Better

1. **Breathing Techniques** use our body's natural breathing response in an intentional way to reduce stress and promote comfort.

2. **Art** can refer to creating something that's visual (like drawings, paintings, etc.), auditory (like musical songs, instrumentals, etc.), written (like poems, stories, etc.), performed (like dance, theater, etc.), interactive (like gardening, cooking, etc.), and more—art is anything that uses imagination to express ideas.

3. **Animal-Assisted Support** can come in different forms and species, but bonding with an animal that brings comfort can help create a feeling of safety.

4. **Cooking** is an artistic expression through food.

5. **Photography** captures images to be shared.

6. **Crafting** is producing something by hand (like knitting, scrapbooking, etc.).

7. **Writing** stimulates the exploration of thoughts through words, ultimately increasing self-awareness and introspection.

8. **Massage** manipulates the body through touch in order to decrease tension.

9. **Mindfulness** is a relaxation strategy that can be used to reduce reactivity and judgement through self-awareness and being present.

10. **Cartooning** combines the visual arts (like drawing, painting, etc.) and writing (like stories, commentaries, etc.) to tell a narrative.

11. Listening to, singing to, moving to, or creating **music** is a positive form of distraction and self-expression.

12. **Filmmaking** is creation of films or videos for story-telling purposes.

13. **Yoga** uses a combination of exercise, breathing techniques, and restorative body postures.

14. **Meditation** can be used to change a state of consciousness to promote emotional well-being through relaxation.

15. **Dance** uses movement as a language for self-expression, incorporating the body, mind, and emotions in an enjoyable way.

16. **Acupuncture** restores natural energy pathways by stimulating specific points of the body using needles.

17. **Guided Imagery** prompts mental images and encourages a full experience of sensory feelings.

18. **Gardening** utilizes self-expression through plants and nature.

19. **Performance Arts** present self-expression through a live act.

20. **Craniosacral Techniques** use gentle touch to put pressure on specific parts of the body in the form of a massage.

21. **Aromatherapy** uses essential oils to send messages to the brain to prompt memories and sensations and can alter your emotions.

22. **Hypnotherapy** uses guided imagery to relax and focus on pleasurable experiences.

23. **Poetry** and **journaling** are ways to express ideas and emotions through words to evoke emotions and thought.

24. **Theater** explores stories and problems through drama, allowing experimentation through interaction and performance.

25. **Pet Training** strengthens the human-animal bond, which can increase the feeling of support, and reduces stress.

26. **Relaxation Strategies** (like breathing exercises, mindfulness, etc.) relieve stress and promote calmness.

27. **Exercise programs** help improve physical activity in a safe manner.

28. **Makeup** is a form of artistic expression on the face or body.

29. **Animation** is the process of directing pictures to have the impression of movement.

30. **Acupressure** is similar to acupuncture without the needles, using pressure to stimulate specific points of the body.

31. **Nail art** is the process of adding artistic details to manicures or pedicures.

32. **Biofeedback** observes your body's activity through sensors and devices that can help to understand your reaction to triggers.

33. **Volunteering** provides a selfless service at no-charge and can offer a larger sense of community and gratitude.

34. **Movement Programs** can help promote activity and condition positive movement patterns.

Think of the above list of 34 items as a menu of options. *What looked good to you?*

1. _____

2. _____

3. _____

4. _____

5. _____

Strengthening the mind/body connection will rewire your brain, leading to pain relief. Does your list include options that **support your mind and your body?** If not, add some more physically active possibilities to your list, too.

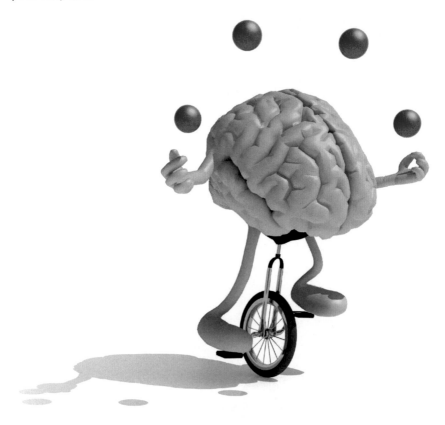

What if you can't do as much movement-wise as you may want to yet? We've all been there! When we reference "physical activity," we are not talking about running a marathon or anything like that. Whatever your final goal is (even if it is running a marathon!), there are <u>steps</u> to get there safely. With chronic pain, you may have cut down on some activities, so just like any other recovery process you start with smaller steps. That's why it's good to create a plan. Let's pick a creative healing option you want to start with.

1. Which creative healing do you want to try?

   _____

2. What is your goal? What are you hoping to accomplish?

   _____

3. What supplies do you need?

   a. Materials: _____

   b. Transportation: _____

   c. Location/Setting: _____

   d. Other: _____

4. Who do you want to do this activity with?

   - Myself

   - Family Member: _____

   - Friend: _____

   - Neighbor: _____

   - Other: _____

5. When are you going to practice this creative healing? For how long?

    Sunday _____

    Monday _____

    Tuesday _____

    Wednesday _____

    Thursday _____

    Friday _____

    Saturday _____

6. How often are you going to have breaks? What will you be doing during your breaks?

    _____

It will be hard to get back into certain activities. While this is challenging, it *can* be done! **Making realistic goals and plans while pacing your activities will help you continue on your path to success.** You may be thinking, "How can something like gardening help with my pain?" Great question!

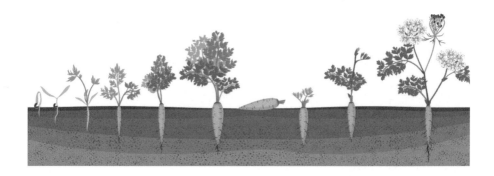

For one thing, gardening usually happens outside. That will help to **motivate** us to get out of the house, which can be enough on some days. It doesn't just get you out of the house, it gets you outside *(which automatically gives you "bonus points")*. In fact, **there is scientific evidence that exposure to nature is therapeutic in itself.** Just being outside exposes your brain to calmness and other good feelings *(the color green actually makes your brain happier unconsciously)*.

While you are gardening, you are moving. Depending on your level of activity, this may include walking around with a hose or watering can *(stamina)*. You may be moving pots or pulling up weeds *(strength)*. You are getting your hands into the soil and feeling the earth under you *(emotional grounding)*. **Movement in any form (while respecting your limits) will help loosen up your muscles and get them used to working again.**

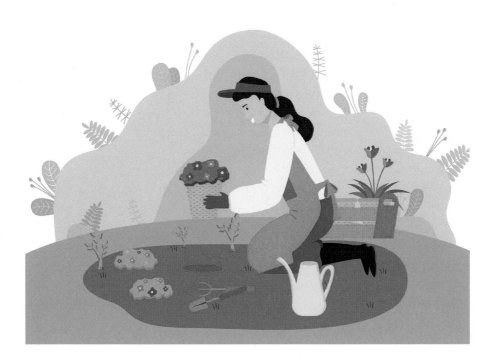

There is also a **creative** and **artistic** side to gardening. What plants do you want to work with? Are they going to be beautiful and delicate like a rose? Or designed with a purpose, like a tomato plant? *Maybe you can do both!* Then, it's a matter of where you want to place them and what the arrangement will look like. What will it look like in a couple of months when it's sprouted? A couple of years? A garden is like nature's canvas. This also goes back to when we were discussing attention. Remember, if we place our attention on something positive and enjoyable *(instead of on the pain),* we can protect our mental garden from pesky predators, *like pain.*

How do you help a garden grow? **Commitment** and **maintenance.** If you don't weed your garden, there will be less room, water, and sunlight for the plants you *do* want. They'll get crowded out. **Choosing a creative healing activity, like gardening, that demands nurturing, will help create a sense of responsibility to keep up your garden.** And by helping your plants sprout, you are growing, too!

Satisfaction in your work is also motivational, and a finished result is a wonderful reward at the end of your hard work. This can be assessed differently depending on the project. Sometimes, fulfillment can come from seeing a rose bud peeking out. Other times you may find it in a jar of homemade, homegrown tomato sauce! Whatever makes you feel proud of your efforts is a prize to enjoy.

Gardening is not for everyone, but it is an excellent example of creative healing and all the dimensions within a practice that can positively affect your well-being. There are even ways to bring nature into your home if you don't have a yard—like indoor plants in pots or windowsill planters! So, in moments of doubt, try breaking up your creative healing like we just did and reminding yourself of all the different benefits it can bring. **Every step that you take, even if it doesn't feel significant, is an extra tool in your kit.**

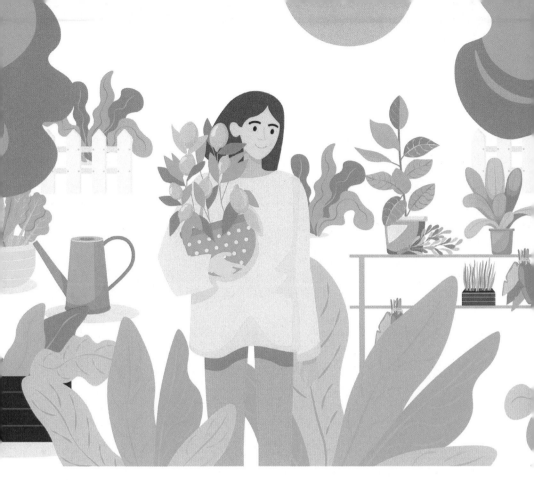

Sometimes you need variety. Not every task can be accomplished by hitting it with a hammer or twisting with a screwdriver. Just like with any preparation, **having options for different problems can be helpful.** So, give some new creative healing strategies a try. You never know what may work for you at different times. **Don't get discouraged if you don't see results right away**—just like a garden takes time to bloom, healing takes time, too. Remember to have a **balance of mind and body strategies, because strengthening your mind/body connection is your best defense against pain resurfacing.**

So, why not start today and reintroduce yourself to your passions?

4c. Who can I turn to for help?

We want to start out by saying, **"You do not 'need' anyone's help."** You are completely capable of arming yourself with tools that can assist with your healing process. Feel free to look back at the last chapter for inspiration at any time! That being said, there is added value to having a support system.

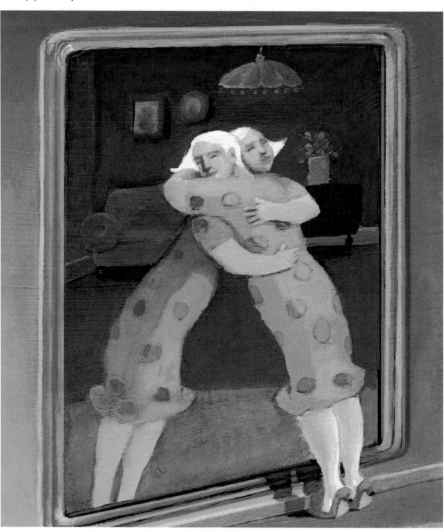

A lot of people with chronic pain turn to a **therapist** for that extra support. Although prioritizing mental health is becoming more widely accepted, there is still hesitancy in certain cultures, communities, and households about going to therapy. We want to reassure you that be-

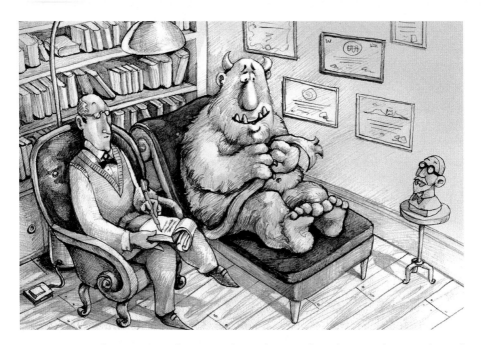

ing prompted to go to a therapist by a doctor, family member, or friend does not mean they think you are "crazy" or that something is "wrong" with you. **Therapy is an opportunity to learn new tools to better deal with your pain,** while also getting to know yourself on a deeper level. *Remember how we keep talking about the mind-body connection and how thoughts, emotions, and feelings impact how the body perceives pain?* Many, **many, <u>many</u>** successful people see therapists regularly and view it as an asset to their self-care!

Similarly, finding the right doctor makes all the difference in the world. Many frequent visitors to doctors' offices or hospitals feel pessimistic about those working in the medical world, but the good ones are out there! Try to find someone who takes the time to get to know you and who sees you as a whole person, rather than a list of symptoms. We also recommend that they have a thorough understanding of chronic pain in children so they come from a place of knowledge and experience when treating you.

Also, take some time thinking about what creative healing strategies are important to you, and then look for someone who can help you experiment. This might be a yoga instructor, music therapist, art therapist, physical therapist, acupuncturist, hypnotherapist, massage therapist …

the list is endless! We recommend making sure these professionals are certified in their scope of practice and that they understand how to work with someone who has chronic pain. Even if there is no one with that specialty in your area, **there are growing opportunities to connect with professionals online in a safe and beneficial way.**

We are well aware that one of our goals in this book is to empower your use of creative healing to modify your overactive nervous system. We cannot skip over medications or dismiss their usefulness. **For certain situations and for some people, medication can be helpful and necessary.** Our intentions are not to "stigmatize" medications or label them as "bad." We would like to encourage you to consider **supplementing your medications** (or whatever Western bio-medical approaches you use) with some creative healing, because they work together. At the end of the day, the whole point is for **you to create your own toolkit** and if medication is one of those tools, then add it in there.

Some of you may have tried a therapist in the past that didn't work out, or you are feeling skeptical of doctors … all of those feelings are valid based on your past experiences. We would still like to encourage you to consider finding the right fit for you, because when you do, it feels so good to have that person in your corner. Just as with certain classmates or teachers you may not click with, the same can be true for members of your treatment team. One "bad apple" should not represent your future relationship with everyone else in that same field.

Don't forget about family, friends, classmates, teachers, teammates, coaches, neighbors, pets—anyone who you think can support you! Think back to who has always had that special talent of making you laugh or who gives you that loving hug when you need a pick-me-up. Sometimes when we feel isolated in our health journey, it can feel strange reaching out to people again.

Where do I even start? Send a short text, write an email, message through social media—send a letter via carrier pigeon! Try doing anything that you can to reignite and/or grow your relationships with loved ones, because you deserve to have a support system. Everyone does.

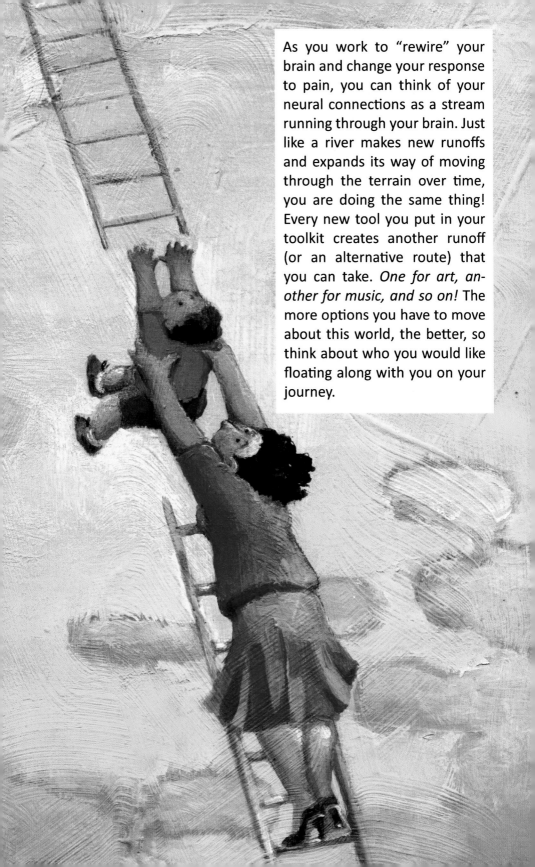

As you work to "rewire" your brain and change your response to pain, you can think of your neural connections as a stream running through your brain. Just like a river makes new runoffs and expands its way of moving through the terrain over time, you are doing the same thing! Every new tool you put in your toolkit creates another runoff (or an alternative route) that you can take. *One for art, another for music, and so on!* The more options you have to move about this world, the better, so think about who you would like floating along with you on your journey.

4d. What did I do wrong? Nothing!

No! You did not do anything wrong. **Your chronic pain is a result of your smart brain trying to protect you.** *So, how can that be "wrong?"* It can't! So now that you know that you can direct your energy toward what you want your brain to learn and enjoy.

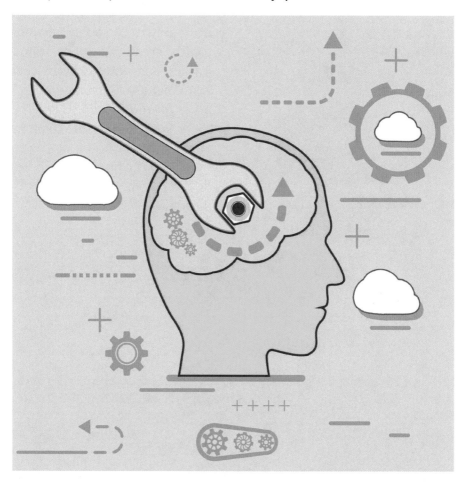

Pain can be a destructive force in your life, like a fire raging across a mountainside. That's why it's important to know how to stop your pain wildfire from spreading, but **it is equally important to know what fuels your pain** so you can remove it from the path. The ammunition for your pain can come in different forms, but it comes down to something called *catastrophizing.*

Have you ever thought something was going to be worse than it ended up being? Here is a common example: *I had a pain flare-up in fourth period yesterday, so that means I may have pain in fourth period today, too. What if the pain gets really bad? What if I can't control it? I don't want to be in pain, so I won't go to school today.*

While we agree that it may feel scary to face the possibility of your pain being triggered, this is *catastrophizing* at its finest. It is your brain trying to protect you. It doesn't want you to feel pain, so it's trying to make sure you do everything you can to avoid it. But, whether your fourth period is geometry, geography, or graphic design, it's important, and you shouldn't be avoiding it.

Your pain may come and go at times. Now that you know the importance of attention, do you see how focusing on the *potential* of having pain in fourth period and spending your energy *(and attention)* worrying about that can start the flow of "bad traffic" and *cause* pain? That is how catastrophizing works—like adding more fuel to the pain fire. Your pain feeds off the *potential* threat *(and fear)* of more pain, leading to more pain and destruction in your life.

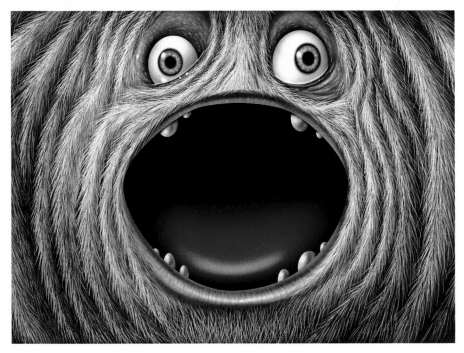

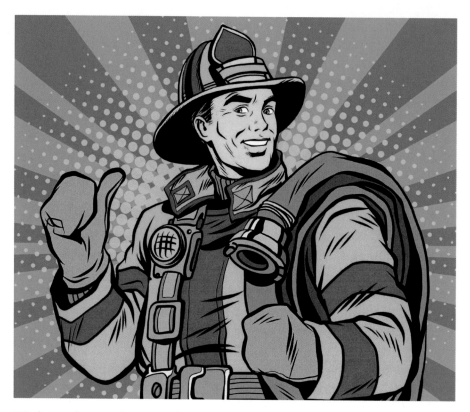

We know how pain spreads—now, how do we stop it in its tracks?

There are multiple ways of snuffing a flame, but what we are talking about is a raging wildfire threatening your happiness and well-being.

Have you ever watched firefighters trying to extinguish a blaze?

1. Excess brush needs to be removed before it becomes new fuel for the wildfire. *This is **your newfound understanding of how pain works in your brain.***

2. Helicopters drop flame-retardant on areas of concern, to prevent the fire from spreading in new directions. *This is **your creative healing that you do to prevent and address pain.***

3. Firefighters and helicopters douse the flames with as much water as they can, trying to eliminate the threat. *This is **your ability keep your attention on the present.***

We know that being "present" is the water that douses our pain wild-fires and prevents them from spreading, but what does that mean? Focusing on the present is about paying attention to what's happening now, instead of worrying about pain you experienced in the past *(ru-minating)* or pain that you imagine in the future *(catastrophizing)*. It brings you back to the moment, which is really the only thing you can directly influence. Some people refer to this skill as *mindfulness.* The past and future are important, but they are out of your control. **You can affect your present and be active in it,** instead of spending your valuable attention on things you can't touch.

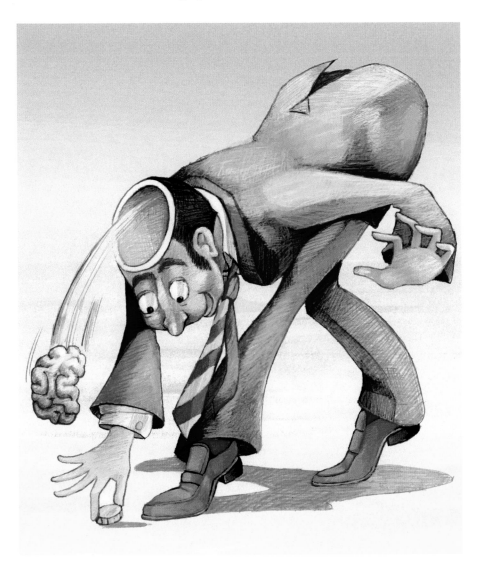

Everyone's mind wanders—thoughts are always popping around and grabbing your attention. Imagine looking at the world through a camera lens. You can see many objects and capture them at one time with the click of a button. But remember, we can only really observe *(and think about)* one thing at a time. So, we want to be intentional with where we aim our brain's camera *and* what we focus it on. Whether it's a snap of a landscape or a portrait of a friend, your camera lens *(and your brain)* needs something to focus on. This is where **mindfulness** comes in.

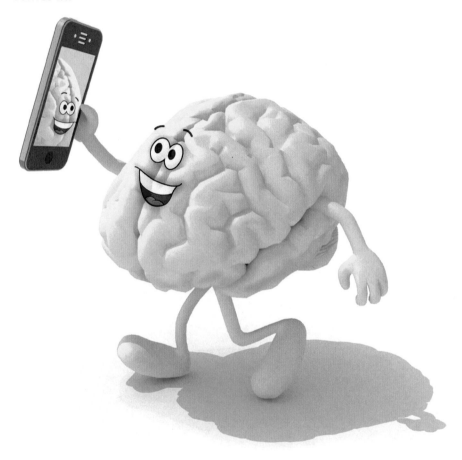

Do you really want to think about how much pain you were in two weeks ago, or about the possibility of pain a year from now? No. You don't *want* to think about that, but you do, and all that really does is cause more distress *(and pain)*. It becomes a self-fulfilling prophecy that no one wants to believe in, but we still kind of do believe in, **so then it becomes true!**

Mindfulness is not about ignoring, because the act of "ignoring" in it-self is placing attention on something you don't want to pay attention to. Like if we asked you not to think about an elephant. Seriously, *DO NOT* think about an elephant. *What is the first thing that popped into your mind?* You probably imagined an elephant! **"Ignoring" just puts more pressure on an already stressful situation.**

If we really don't want you to think about an elephant, we shouldn't ask you to ignore it. Instead, we should suggest a different thought—**something else to place your attention on,** because with your smart brain, simply expecting the absence of a thought is just not going to cut it.

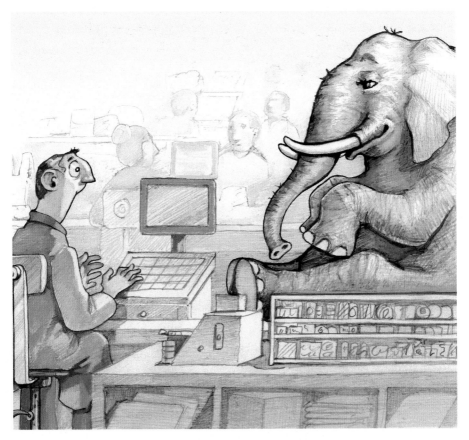

Now, we want you to think about a rose. Imagine the blush pink and soft petals gently folding over themselves. Picture a few drops of that morning's dew still perched on the surface, close to rolling off, but still hugging the flower closely. *Can you smell its perfume?*

What are you thinking about now? If even for just a moment an elephant was not occupying your mind, then you can see how mindfulness works. Let's go back to an elephant for another quick example. There is an old parable that originated in India. Since it has so much history and it has spread to many cultures, the exact story and meaning varies, but here is one general version in a nutshell:

A group of blind men came across an elephant. They had never encountered an elephant before, so they had no idea what it was. Since they could not study it visually, they had to observe it through touch. Each person reached out and caressed a part of the elephant. One stroked the long, flexible trunk and one handled the thick, sturdy leg. Another found the hard, sharp ivory tusk, and one of the men felt the rough skin along the elephant's rib cage. *Maybe one person even got tickled by the swish of the friendly tail!*

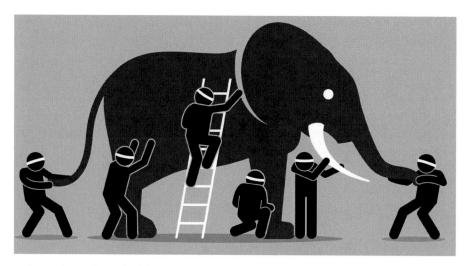

When they described what they felt, each man had a completely different explanation of their experience of the same animal. And each description was right! Each person was working with the reality that they were exposed to. They just didn't have a complete illustration of the entire mammal.

Like the elephant, the story is open to interpretation, and so is your experience. Each person experiences life in their own subjective way. Absolutely everything is subjective based on personal experience—even something that seems as concrete as "truth."

So, back to the title of this chapter: **Did I do anything wrong?**

No.

No.

No. No! No!!!!

What you did, and what you will continue to do, is **move through your life based on your personal experiences.** If you are reading this book out of order or skipped to this chapter, this is not our version of saying "the pain is in your head." **You were (or are) feeling pain. That is the truth.**

Just like the blind men who understood what an elephant was, based on what they knew to be true, **you learned your response to pain based on what you knew to be true.** *But there is good news!* Learning is a process, and the fact that you are still curious and motivated to absorb all this means that you now have the ability to piece it all together!

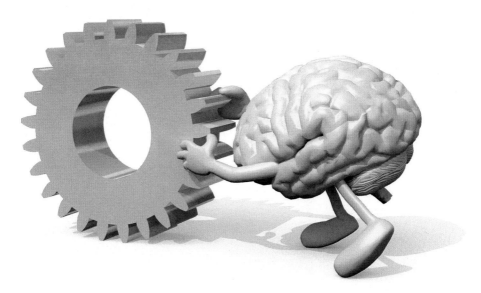

Now, you have the choice to move through your life the way you have been, or you can choose to know there are other parts of the elephant that you haven't discovered yet and **purposefully enjoy the process of that discovery.**

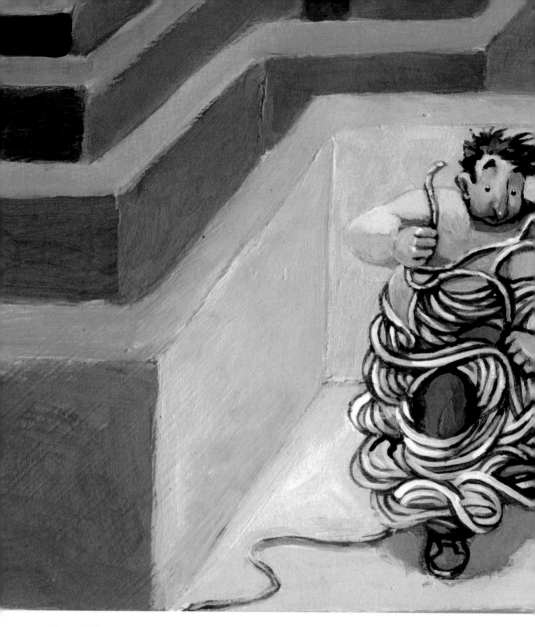

4e. When will my pain go away?

The truth is, we don't have the answer to this question. We wish we did, but we don't.

It's not as simple as taking a pill twice a day or wearing a cast for six weeks. Rewiring your brain to heal your mind and body is no easy feat, but it has been done—and you can do it, too!

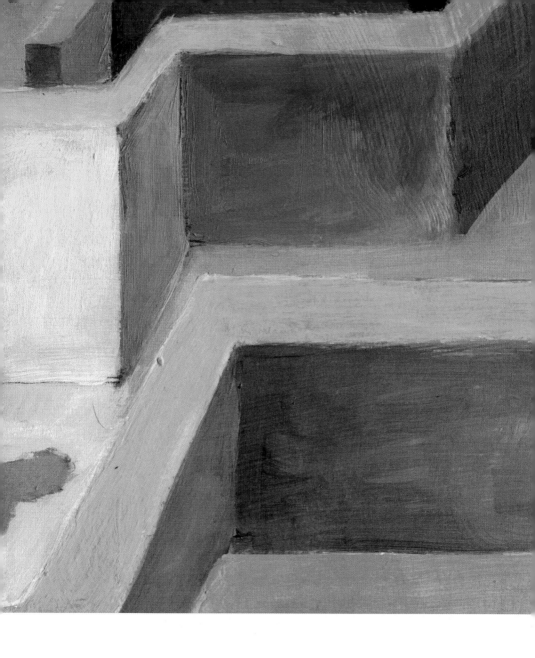

The "good" news about having this kind of Smart Brain Pain Syndrome while you're young is that **your brain is accustomed to learning.** This is called *neuroplasticity,* meaning the younger the brain, the more flexible it is. This flexibility gives you the ability to reorganize your brain, teaching it to work the way you *want* it to.

Many people ask, "What should I do first?" Just as a personal trainer at the gym can't give one set of instructions suitable for every single person's workout routine, we can't suggest a universal first step either. And it's probably not your first step, or your second, your third, or your eleventh! We encourage you to do what is *doable* for you. **The goal is to regulate and get your nervous system back into balance from the brain down.**

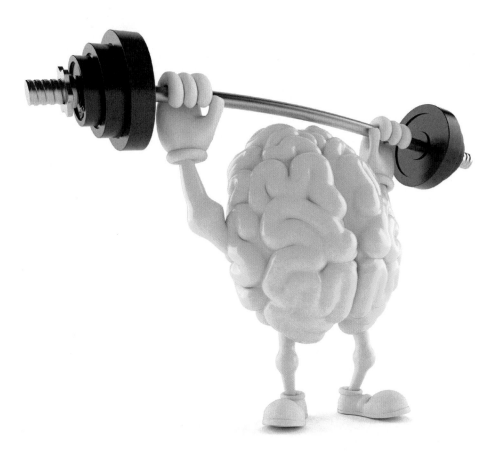

Odds are that if you've been in pain, you have not been as active as you would like to be. Since you're in pain and are not moving as much, your muscles could become fatigued more easily. Then, when you try to work those muscles that are already tired, this causes more pain. And so, you don't want to move as much. *It's a vicious cycle!* If you haven't used something in a while, it can be difficult to start up again.

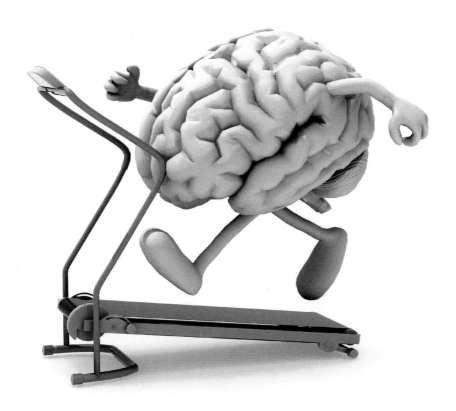

Just like going to the gym to strengthen your body and practice new ways of working it, you need to consistently go to the "brain gym," too. The more you use your creative healing, the more opportunity you have to send positive messages from the mind to the body—and also from the body to the mind. **This multi-directional dialogue can only be accomplished through practice and goes back to the wellness balance that we all hope to achieve.**

When your body gets out of balance, it can feel like you're stuck in a snowball rolling down a freshly powdered mountain. As you rumble down the slope, every rotation makes your snowball bigger and heavier so it falls down even faster! Every time you don't get a good night's sleep, miss school, or get into an argument with a friend, your snowball grows and rolls, until you're at the bottom of the hill looking up at what seems like Mount Everest. *How the heck am I going to get to the top again?* It seems impossible.

Not to worry, though, even if you are at the foot of what seems like a cliff. As each layer of ice melts, you become freer from the constraints of your snowball. When you no longer have the cold, wetness, and discomfort *(pain)* to focus your attention on, you are still stuck looking up at this huge, intimidating mountain.

It is not easy to climb a mountain, and it won't be accomplished in a day. It takes work. Little by little, you can hike for a few hours, hit an icy patch, and slide back down a bit. But you have to get back up and look at where you've come from! Maybe you are still a third of the way up the mountain. **So, you keep working and working until eventually you get to the top.** And wow, that is a pretty view!

Do you know who will make it to the top of a mountain like chronic pain? It is not about who has the strongest muscles or the most expensive hiking gear. The way to measure if someone will make it or not is based on one word: **resilience.**

Resilience is broad, yet specific. It does not have any precise requirements. To put it simply, **resilience is having the will and ability to keep going, no matter what.**

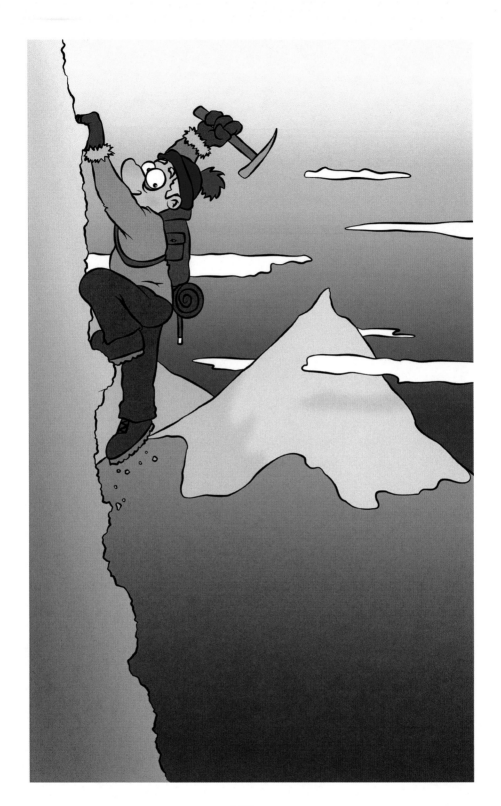

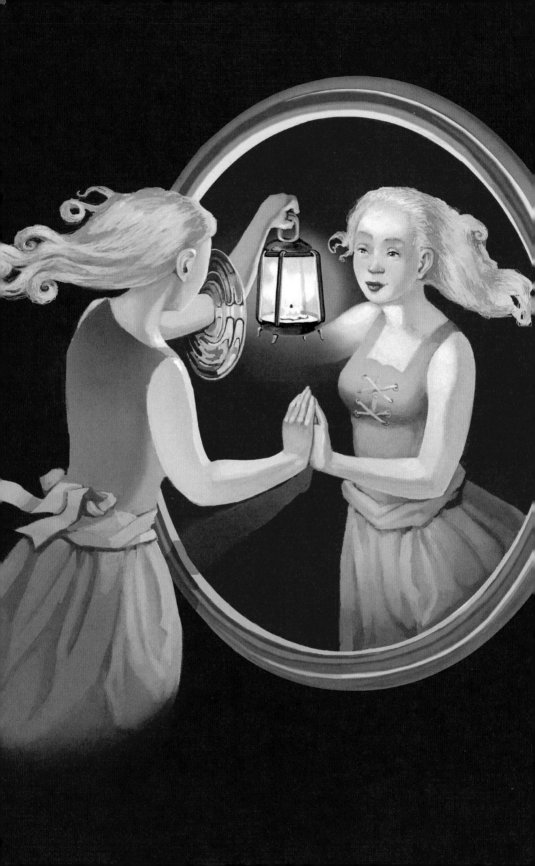

You can build resilience out of the skills learned from creative healing. And, once you've gained resilience **there's no time limit on it.** Yours will come, and when it does you will know you are resilient. You probably don't know you are resilient until it happens. It's like a superpower that you didn't know you had until one day (when you really need it), it came out to show you that **you can do the work and succeed.**

Just like anything good in life, you have to earn resilience on your own (through the act of doing). Once you've *done* **it**—once you have unleashed your resilience and are able to maintain it—**absolutely no person or thing can take it away from you.**

Resilience is the ultimate tool in life, that can and will get you wherever you *want* **to go.**

Hopefully after reading this book, you feel more empowered to get what you want and deserve for your healing process.

You have what it takes. You are strong enough to do this. Your body and brain can work together to lessen the presence of pain in your life. The greatest thing that you can do is to trust and honor yourself. Let yourself be your guide.

The moral of the story is—this is YOUR story. You may not have a bunch of fancy diplomas on your wall (yet!) but even right now, in this moment, you are the expert on your pain.

Use this link to find pediatric pain programs in the U.S. and Canada:

http://childpain.org/wp-content/uploads/2021/01/Pediatric-Chronic-Pain-Programs-2021-Update.pdf

Want to learn more about your brain and pain? Visit *mychyp.org* and look around our growing Resource Library. Here are some great videos to get you started:

- *https://www.aboutkidshealth.ca/pain*
- *https://www.retrainpain.org/*
- *https://www.tamethebeast.org/*
- *https://www.youtube.com/watch?v=C_3phB93rvI*
- *https://www.youtube.com/watch?v=J6--CMhcCfQ*
- *https://www.aci.health.nsw.gov.au/chronic-pain/painbytes*

Creative Healing for Youth in Pain (CHYP) is a nonprofit providing educational resources, social support, and exposure to creative healing experiences for youth with chronic pain and their parents online. Our virtual format allows us to connect families with our services regardless of geographic location, socioeconomic status, insurance status, race, ethnicity, and more. To learn more about the organization and our current programs, please visit *www.mychyp.org* or follow us on social media:

Instagram: *@my_chyp*
Twitter: *@my_chyp*
Facebook: Creative Healing for Youth in Pain
YouTube: Creative Healing for Youth in Pain
Email: *admin@mychyp.org*

CHYP is a 501(c)3 nonprofit. If you are interested in making a tax-deductible donation, please visit: *www.mychyp.org/donate*

More by the authors:

Pain in Children & Young Adults: The Journey Back to Normal, by Lonnie Zeltzer, MD, & Paul Zeltzer, MD

The Drs. Zeltzers offer specific strategies to take control of the pain—regardless of cause(s). The book guides you in understanding pain in general as well as specific pain conditions and explores how children express pain, along with how to interpret what they say. The authors provide sage advice from top pain professionals in the world.

Vienna's Waiting, by Georgia Huston Weston

An intensely personal journey of anguish, solitude, and despair.

At 14, Georgia was on top of the world. Her life as a teenager was filled with hope and promise, until a mysterious pain developed in her back and legs. When doctors failed to help, she spiraled into hopelessness. This book chronicles her feelings during that dark period of her life and follows her inspirational journey back to health and happiness. *(Also available as an audiobook.)*

PAIN: An Owner's Manual, by Georgia Huston Weston

If you hurt, read this book! A young pain victim's inspirational and informative conversations with a variety of pain sufferers and specialists. They share their experiences with pain, their coping strategies, and what works for them in getting through the day.

Astonishingly frank conversations range from marijuana use to childbirth to suicide. A must-read for all doctors, who will get an earful from the other side of the examination room. Different therapies and coping strategies work for different people. There are realistic discussions of therapies such as biofeedback, Iyengar yoga, and hypnotherapy. Horror stories turn into hopeful tales of personal heroism, perseverance, family unity, and caring.

Doctors should read this at their own risk.

Thank you to CHYP's team of volunteers (past and present)!

Board of Directors
Risë Barbakow; Tina Bryson, PhD, LCSW; Maya Iwanaga Pinkner, JD; Julia Kelly; Cindy McCann; Dana Pachulski; Beth Wishnie; Lonnie Zeltzer, MD

Clinical Advisory Board Members
Sarah Ahola Kohut, PhD, CPsych; Rachael Coakley, PhD; Sabine Combrie, PT, CST; Elizabeth Donovan, PhD; Liatt Granott; Anya Griffin, PhD; Elliott Krane, MD; Rona Levy, MSW, PhD, MPH; Samantha Levy, PhD; Sarah Martin, PhD; Mariela Nava, DNP, CPNP; Diane Poladian, PT, DPT, OCS; Tonya Palermo, PhD; Neil Schechter, MD; Shelley Segal, PsyD; Soumitri Sil, PhD; Rachel Zoffness, PhD

Arts Council Members
Cory Hills, Anatalia Hordov, Daniel Leighton, Nina Mathews, MFT, Ted Meyer, Dominic Quagliozzi, Wellington (PJ) Smith

Volunteers
Naomi Abergel, Nadia Ansari, Olivia Aviera, Parth Bhatt, Sara Castle, Laura Cavanagh, Antonin Combrie, Maggie Fuzak, Madison Goon, Marisa Holt, MFT, Layan Kaileh, Matthew Kuan, Bertha Lopez, Jonathan Pachulski, Nicola Pachulski, Chyna Parker, Lydia Schinasi, Hannah Selesnick, Holly Scott-Gardner, Trozalla Smith, Rebecca Stein, ASW, Kayla Taft, Katherina Tanson, Hannah Zelcer

Cover artwork by Alexandra Castle.

A special thanks to Scott Bryson, Jimmy Huston, Lynn Mills, Veronica Huston, and Cosworth Publishing for their expert editing and production.

Sponsored by Whole Child LA

Lonnie Zeltzer, M.D., is a Distinguished Research Professor of Pediatrics, Anesthesiology, Psychiatry, and Biobehavioral Sciences at the David Geffen School of Medicine at UCLA and Immediate Past-Director for 30 years of the UCLA Pediatric Pain and Palliative Care Program. She is a co-author on the Institute of Medicine report on Transforming Pain in America and was an invited member of the national steering committee assigned to provide directions for pain research at the National Institutes of Health (NIH).

Dr. Zeltzer has received, among other awards, a Mayday Pain and Policy Fellowship and the 2005 Jeffrey Lawson Award for Advocacy in Children's Pain Relief from the American Pain Society (APS). Her UCLA integrative pediatric pain program received a 2009 Clinical Centers of Excellence in Pain Management Award from APS and a 2012 award from the Southern California Cancer Pain Initiative. She is active in advocacy for pain care and research, and was an invited member of the Centers for Disease Control (CDC) Special Advisor on The State of Opioids in America.

In addition, she is an invited member of the FDA Committee on Analgesia and Anesthesia Products, where new pain-related drugs are given FDA approval or not, as well as an invited member of the Expert Advisory Committee on Hemoglobinopathies as a pain expert for the National Heart, Lung, and Blood Institute (NHLBI) at NIH. She is also on an expert panel for the NIH on a national study on a mind-body intervention for teens with fibromyalgia, and is a member of the national Autism Think Tank as a pain expert in autism.

Dr. Zeltzer's research includes yoga, mindfulness, hypnotherapy, and other self-help interventions, including mobile technologies, to help children and adolescents who have chronic pain, as well as understanding biopsychosocial pain mechanisms in irritable bowel syndrome, cancer, sickle cell disease, headaches, dysmenorrhea, and other conditions. She has over 350 research publications on childhood pain and complementary therapies, has written more than 80 chapters, and published her first book for parents on chronic pain in childhood (Harper-Collins, 2005) and her second book for parents on chronic pain in children and young adults (Shilysca Press, 2016). Dr. Zeltzer is the Founder and President of Creative Healing for Youth in Pain (*www.mychyp.org*).

Paul Zeltzer, M.D., Co-Director of WCLA Inc., joins the clinical team with expertise in diagnosis and management of pain in children with cancer and blood diseases. He is Board-Certified in Pediatrics & Hematology and Oncology.

He developed and directed clinical investigations for leukemia and brain tumors with the National Cancer Institute and private industry clinical trials, as well as editing major textbooks in Oncology and Neurooncology. He published over 130 publications studying molecular biology, treatment results, and long term outcomes of cancer treatment. He is an advisor and supports more than five pediatric and adult cancer websites. He is a Clinical Professor in Neurosurgery, Geffen School of Medicine, University of California at Los Angeles.

Dr. Zeltzer has authored books for the lay public: *Brain Tumors: Leaving the Garden of Eden* (2004) and *Brain Tumors: Finding the Ark* (2006). Both are #1, 2 in their niche category. In 2016, he coauthored with Dr. Lonnie Zeltzer: *Pain in Children and Young Adults: The Journey Back to Normal.* He has given medical advice to several television series, including "The Bold Ones" (1969-1970) and "SCRUBS" (2002-2008).

As an inventor, he has two approved US patents: System and Method for Storing Information on a Wireless Device. The GoMed Application (US patent 6,970,827B2 11-10-2005) and United States Patent 10,278,725 May 7, 2019 Lumbar puncture detection device—an improved LP needle.

Drs. Paul and Lonnie Zeltzer are co-Directors of Whole Child LA (*www. wholechildla.com*), a clinic for children and young adults with complicated chronic pain.

Georgia Weston, LCSW, is the Executive Director of Creative Healing for Youth in Pain (CHYP), a nonprofit that provides educational resources, creative healing experiences, and social support for youth with chronic pain and their parents. (*www.mychyp.org*)

Georgia has a Bachelor of Arts in psychology, with a minor in art, from St. Edward's University. She has a Master of Social Work degree from the University of Southern California, with a concentration in Children, Youth, and Families, as well as a focus in Child and Adolescent Mental Health. She is a Licensed Clinical Social Worker.

She has experience creating and leading programs for organizations that provide therapeutic services for struggling individuals and families. She also has clinical social work experience, both as an outpatient therapist and residential therapist, for youth dealing with complex cognitive, behavioral, and social needs. And, she has been a Research Associate with the UCLA Pediatric Pain Research Program.

The author of two books, *Vienna's Waiting* and *PAIN: An Owner's Manual,* she provides insight into the mysterious world of chronic pain through her own story and the stories of others.

In 2011, she founded the Teen Pain Help Foundation (*www.teenpainhelp.org*), a 501(c)3 charitable corporation created to help children and adolescents with chronic pain. Since then Georgia has served as the Executive Director, raising funds for treatment, research, education, and increased public awareness of pediatric chronic pain. She also co-founded and was the Director of Programming for Art Rx, strengthening the partnership between the USC Suzanne Dworak-Peck School of Social Work and the USC Keck School of Medicine, specifically to better understand how art impacts pain.

In recognition of her humanitarian services, Georgia received the David Chow Humanitarian Foundation Award for 2019. Georgia is dedicated to empowering youth with chronic pain, and their families, through creative healing techniques and social support.

Reviews

"Awesome, a book for young people with pain that comes from a such a good place. By combining experience with expertise, this leading team have organized the right material in the right way, and delivered it with aplomb, with empathy, and with skill. If you are struggling to make sense of why pain is still there, struggling to find the right words or pictures, or just need to know that there are others in the world who understand, then this is for you."
Christopher Eccleston, PhD - Professor of Medical Psychology, and Director of the Centre for Pain Research at the University of Bath, UK.

"Smart Brain Pain Syndrome is a terrific resource for teens struggling with chronic pain. The authors bring decades of clinical experience treating (and living with) complex chronic pain, and readers will benefit from the wisdom they convey with warmth, positivity, and encouragement. Through the use of metaphors and humor, the book presents complex scientific constructs in language that is accessible and appealing. Smart Brain Pain Syndrome will help young chronic pain sufferers truly understand and embrace the mind-body connection and develop a personalized set of creative healing tools to help them take back their lives."
Deirdre Logan, PhD - Director of Psychology Services in Pain Medicine; Department of Anesthesia, Boston Children's Hospital; Associate Professor, Harvard Medical School

"This is a brilliant handbook for teens coping with chronic pain. The use of metaphors, examples, and explanations of pain and the mind-body connection are simple but sophisticated. This is an engaging resource that teens will find motivating as they learn to incorporate creative healing strategies into their toolbox for coping with chronic pain."
Tonya Palermo, PhD - Professor of Anesthesiology, Adj. Pediatrics and Psychiatry, University of Washington; Hughes M. and Katherine Blake Endowed Professorship in Health Psychology; Associate Director, Center for Child Health Behavior and Development, Seattle Children's Research Institute

"As educators, we often have students who struggle to engage in learning due to the impact of chronic pain. The information presented in The Smart Brain Pain Syndrome provides clarity in the "why" behind the pain as well as a plethora of solutions that can be incorporated in a school-based plan to support a student's academic and social emotional success within the school setting. We highly recommend this book to all educators as an important resource!"
Carin, Marine, and Sandy @theintentionalprincipal

Made in United States
Orlando, FL
20 June 2022

18997004R00075